WALK
LIKE A MAN

WALK LIKE A MAN

A FAMILY'S WALK WITH CLAY AND HIS WALK WITH BEING GAY AND LIVING WITH AIDS

Ann Baker

Writers Club Press

San Jose New York Lincoln Shanghai

WALK LIKE A MAN
A family's walk with Clay
And his walk with being gay and living with AIDS

Writers Club Press
an imprint of iUniverse.com, Inc.

For information address:
iUniverse.com, Inc.
5220 S 16th, Ste. 200
Lincoln, NE 68512
www.iuniverse.com

ISBN: 0-595-20159-8

Printed in the United States of America

Dedication

For years I have been saying "as soon as this is over, I'm going to write a book". Well, it's over..at least the physical part...and the walk has been long and hard.

Clay, my second son, and I discussed writing a book for years. I'm sure his version would have been much different. I wanted him to write his own story: finding out he was gay, his feelings, and his experiences while traveling, his life in California, his experiences with the new gay disease. He never did. He just lived it. His actions, his activities, and his contributions to the world are telling their own story of his life.

Then I realized Clay's story is a story about Clay, as a person, and me, as a person, and the people in our paths.

I chose the title "Walk Like A Man" for reasons that will become obvious as the story unfolds.

This book is dedicated to Clay, who was "a mixed blessing", and to the bodies strewn along the path of the epidemic called AIDS hewn out of history. It is my hope and the hope of those who knew and loved Clay that our experience will make someone else's walk less painful, less lonely.

The words and the spirit of this book are dedicated to the unselfish, loving people who walked with Clay in Long Beach, Oklahoma City, Tahlequah and Norman, Oklahoma. It is an attempt to express my thanks to those souls who allowed Clay to walk with dignity during those long last days: first of all my children, Matt, Dan and his wife, Shelly, Annie and her friend, Van, Woody, Dave, James and Jane, Gloria, Sarah, Eck, Ron T., Louise and Bill, Tim, Nick, Mary, Marty, Owana,

Ron and Bonnie, Steve and Monya, Harold, Leslie, the staff of Jeffrey Beal's office in Tulsa, the Home Health Care people in Tahlequah, Oklahoma, the angels who sat with Clay during the last days at St. John's Hospital, and, of course, his precious dogs, Annabelle and Camille. And, my grateful thanks to God for his protection and grace during long, impossible days and nights.

Thank you all for your love, caring and support.

Contents

THE BEGINNING

Every little boy is probably told at one time or another: "stand up and be a man" or "act like a man" or "someday you'll be a man". These are worthy admonitions and can provide a road map, if the persons giving the advice, the role models, and the person receiving the advice have the same definition of "a man".

I can give my definition of a "man" at this point in my own life…more so the family of man, who are those humans who share the planet with one another. When I was young, a new wife, a young, impressionable and dysfunctional (by some standards) woman and mother, I thought a "man" was a male who protected his family, loved and cherished his mate, worked hard to earn a living, was polite and respectful to women, loved and played with his children. In short, I had unrealistic expectations of another person, of marriage, husbands, men, fathers, my family and myself.

I married young, learned some hard lessons very quickly, gave birth to two lively, intelligent sons whose father was a man who was completely self-absorbed with his manly activities and unaware of our little family's need for care and support. I did not realize what was wrong and found a way to extricate myself and my children from the reality of what that "man" perceived as a "marriage". I blamed the man.

Immediately, I jumped into a second relationship and eventually married an older man who seemed to be the opposite of my first husband. He was affectionate, concerned and caring, the very attributes I was craving.

I was convinced we had the kind of love which would last forever. He was divorced after a long marriage and had two pre-teen children who were being coached by their mother to believe that their new step-mother was the epitome of evil.

I was undaunted by the combined problems of acceptance by the stepchildren, the emotional effect my divorce had on my own babies, and the complete opposition to my decisions by my family. God had given me a partner who would fill that yet unidentified void in my life. Upward and onward was my theme. I proceeded to throw myself into making my new husband totally happy. I began to put a new family together. I knew in my mind and heart that our love could overcome all problems......past, present, and future. It did not occur to me that what "I" could do was sorely limited by my inexperience and immaturity and by true life situations.

My sons were only two and three at the time of my divorce and second marriage. I had rationalized that the transition would be less painful at this young age than later in life. Being a child of a "broken" marriage and a pretty unsettled home life afterwards, I was living in my own little dream world. I had no idea what a relationship truly entailed. I had no experience with interacting with another human in a give-and-take manner. I did all the giving and did it willingly and lovingly. The philosophy of marriage, of two people in building a life together as a united front, but as two separate beings, never was a part of my living process. I was clueless about motherhood, and did not know it.

As a product of a family who did not show affection or exhibit nurturing, and a family riddled with alcoholism, I did not know how to love without suffocating. I did not know how a mother and a father, a wife and a husband were supposed to function in order to provide stepping stones for the children to learn and develop in a healthy, happy way.

I can only quote an often-used, maudlin well-meaning phrase: "I did the best with what I had to work with". We all did. I was 49 years old before I realized that I did not function properly and that my children, husbands, my whole family, even myself had suffered needlessly because of my lack of insight into my own dysfunction.

Not that our lives were so bad. My second husband and I were married nearly 18 years. My first two sons, and then our son and daughter, and even his children, had many good times. We were able to do all the family things and had nice homes in both the city and the country. The kids had dogs and cats and rabbits and pet squirrels. They hunted, fished, had creeks and rivers to play around, were active in Sunday School and church, Cub Scouts, Brownies, Girl Scouts, baseball, choir, football, swimming and drama. In other words, they were normal, healthy children. I baked, cooked, gardened, and played with them all. We worked hard for our family, loved doing it and loved the children…the best we knew how.

Each child was unique! I really had thought raising kids would be a snap. All I had to do was love and care for them, and everyone would be happy and well equipped for life. I didn't know our little family was a microcosm of the world. Those four precious little human beings each contained a very different packet of cultural, physical, intellectual, emotional and spiritual attributes. I was in shock as these differences developed and each child responded to our efforts to raise them in completely different ways.

During these "family" years, my husband, as the "man" of the family, thought that he was the master by virtue of his title of husband and father. His perception of that role of master dictated that all of the children should be and act in the manner he expected. I did not realize that this was a little out of kilter. I went along with this method of family raising unaware that there should have been more give and take. This type of family structure and belief was common during the 50's and 60's. It is still a prevalent philosophy in many families and probably works if all of the parameters are "just right". My personal observation is that this type of absolute power often tends to overlook the rights and innate differences of the individuals the family. That's how it worked in our family.

The children tried to "be" what their father and stepfather expected. I pushed and prodded them to conform and obey. Thank God, each child developed in spite of our stumbling efforts to control them. Each began the search for his own identity. Like all human beings, they were on the path to determining where they fit in this world. Each encountered and dealt with experiences which helped them determine that identity sexually, physically, spiritually, mentally and emotionally. They walked different paths, developed different interests and friendships. Each dreamed his own dream. We did not realize just how different one child would be and how his search would affect everyone.

All of the events leading up to this time were "family oriented" and not in reality geared to the individuals who made up the family. And all of these events lead us to my second son, the central figure in this tale…well, maybe not the central figure, but certainly the catalyst that kept our family members in turmoil..the irritant that spurred people to action..positive and negative. This walking, talking enigma was Clay. He paid a hard price for being unique, for his interpretation of how to "walk like a man". He challenged most people's perceptions of their own sets of values. His actions and beliefs caused each of us to examine our own actions and beliefs. We were very reluctant to make these changes. Change was a long time coming. Ultimately, after much struggle and pain, we realize the changes were to our benefit. But, I'm getting ahead of the story. Let's talk about Clay.

Clay was born with big, blue eyes. He was blond, healthy, pleasant and curious. He and his big brother grew up hugging each other. These innocent children stayed right with me as I stumbled through life thinking I was doing the right thing. They took the abuse, accepted the criticism, and struggled to discover what they could do that would be acceptable to the men in their lives… their biological father and their stepfather. When they were five and six, they welcomed with joy the addition of our third son and three years later the birth of their sister.

All of the children were healthy and happy with wonderful minds! But Clay's amazing intellect really became evident when he began school. His ability to comprehend and learn set him apart from other children. From my observation and my conversations with him, this intellectual prowess made him feel "different". He viewed life and the world around him in a light somewhat different from most little boys. He was a little more aesthetic, loved music and art, was tender about the treatment and mistreatment of animals…just enough to be teased by some of the men in his life. He was by no means a sissy, but began developing a great dislike for bullies and tough guys and from an early age could not tolerate inequities.

It was confusing to all of us that Clay was so dissatisfied and critical…not of his brothers and sisters, but of the adults..the way the world was being run. I know he hated me for not understanding and making it "all better"..which I would gladly have done if I were God. He did not accept our way of life. He chose his own religion, friends, music, books,not uncommon in adolescence. We could not do anything right in his eyes. He told me that he thought he had been born into the wrong family.

He thought he should have been born into wealth, and hated our "bourgeois" life.

THE DIFFERENCE

One of the worst parts of being the "survivor" is looking back and wondering why we didn't have the instincts or knowledge to move in closer to this person, to help him work with this feeling of alienation, to rejoice in his uniqueness..WITH HIM. But, this was nearly 20 years ago, in the innocent years..our and his..the world's. We had no idea to what proportions this difference, this uniqueness..would affect Clay's life, our lives, millions of lives. I also wonder now if we were not also dealing with a "manic depressive" condition. In later years, I remember that Clay had mentioned that a counselor had suggested that he might have this disorder. Because we thought we were dealing with a rebellious child, we chose to ignore this suggestion. I wonder how this story would have turned out if we had followed up on this suggestion?

A question I have been asked on a consistent basis is, "How did you feel when you found out your son was gay?" Personally I was very sad for Clay, because I knew that life was tough enough with the stigma of being homosexual. At the time he was waging a battle against his stepfather, and vice versa. I guess he was just RAGING! He was an adolescent. Adolescents rebel! He was bored with our rural life. He wanted excitement! The juices of life and the lure of the world were pulling on him. He chose the wild side, and enjoyed it! We were part of an age-old, universal story...and he thought he was being different.

While Clay was being very difficult and making life miserable for everyone in his path, his older brother was working hard. He was a model student and son. He became a peacemaker. Clay's younger brother and sister were busy growing up, enjoying being young, pretty much ignoring the battles. Despite outward appearances, all of the children were suffering from the fact that Clay was depriving them of their own special time in the family by demanding so much time and energy. They all were struggling to stay clear of the trouble and avoid any additional conflict. Clay was making enough trouble for all of us.

Trouble was truly "a brewin'". I had gone back to work full time about the time Clay started getting out of control. He was "sweet 16". My husband went into an ill-fated business venture. The more I worked, made friends at work, and expanded my world, the more fragmented our married life became. Still trying to be "supermom", I could not pay enough attention or stroke the ego of my husband enough. He found a diversion, which I have since learned that all my boys knew about for several months before I did.

All of these things were fermenting one awful winter when Clay pushed the limits and , as he was so adept at doing, forced us into action. We had given him a choice: obey the rules or leave home. He had really broken so many rules and had become so defiant and abusive that we had to lay down the law. We had other children to care for and to protect.

My husband had told me that the only reason he allowed Clay to stay was because he knew how much I cared. "But," he said, "the first time that boy says anything to you or hurts you, he's out." When he heard Clay tell me to "fuck off", that was it. I no longer was in control of Clay's life. My husband had to take over and treat Clay like a man. If he could not accept the rules of our home and respect his mother, he could go out and fight the world.

The real nightmare began that night. At a little over 16 years of age, this brilliant, talented child was thrown out into the coldest winter our area of the country had experienced in years. My heart nearly broke. I continually worried about him. I watched the news to be sure the body found along the highway,—the newest murder—was not my Clay. Fortunately, a family in a nearby town took him in and helped him get through high school. This family had its own problems and went through some difficult times with Clay, but they protected him for a time. I have always been grateful that they helped.

Clay dropped the bomb on me in about 1976 when he quietly and tearfully told me he was gay. I cannot say I was surprised, but I can say my heart grieved. I grieved for the alienation he was facing, for the loss of his innocence, for the loss of our expectations and dreams we had for each of our children. My heart broke for the devastation this would bring upon his relationships, particularly his father...for the sheer agony he was going through. We had no idea what hell was in store for him...for all of us.

During the next three years my marriage deteriorated. We moved further out in the country to make my husband happy. My stepfather who had helped raise me died. My eldest son graduated from high school, met a girl in college, married her, and became a father. My second marriage finally succumbed to the apparent loss of love, respect and companionship so necessary to hold a family together against the temptations and pressures of everyday life. At about the same time I filed for divorce, my married son who had dropped out of college to take care of wife, stepchildren and a new baby, called in confusion and turmoil to tell me his wife had left him found another more interesting man, and told him he was boring.

What a time! A family in distress. Not a new scenario in the 70's and 80's..but definitely a complicated picture. I now had a divorced son. I was a divorced mother trying to raise a nearly-teen daughter, to soothe Danny, my third son, left with his father and smarting from what he perceived as desertion, and a gay son adrift in the world.

Clay returned when I bought my little house in town. We all tried to live together: Matt, my eldest, Clay, and Annie, my young teenage daughter. When the boys saw I was not going to wash and cook, they

deserted like rats on a sinking ship. Like many children in the same circumstances, it seemed they thought that if my husband (the bad guy at
that time) was not there, everything would be perfect. They would have
their mother all to themselves. However, I was intent on having a good
time for a change. I did all of the things newly single people did. Some
of these activities were not always blessed by society…but it felt good to
me. Hmmm. I wonder where my children developed the propensity for
developing habits that made them feel good? My sons were smart
enough to realize that living with me was not a good idea at the time.
They were wise enough and independent enough to forge their own
trails.

In early 1981, after trying some college and living in Tulsa for a while,
Clay decided to head for Los Angeles, the destination for many young
gay men and women. These were years of very little communication. A
word here and there. I missed him terribly and prayed and prayed for
his safety and happiness. None of us knew anything about the gay
lifestyle and habits. I was hopeful that Clay was living the life he wanted
and confident that he had found a niche for himself. Only later did I
know the truth.

A particularly sad day was telling Clay "good-bye" at the Tulsa airport
in 1981..not knowing we would not see him again until 1986. The "au
revoir" party remains as one of my silliest memories. Clay gave all of us
"silly" memories, moments to make us chuckle and shake our heads. He
and his friends were sure they were on their way to discovering a new
world in which they could express themselves freely. It would be all
good times. They would be with people who understood their needs
and passions. They would be unfettered by convention and the mores of
the Bible belt. Clay was not the only member of the family with this
type of sense of humor. We are all guilty of enjoying a "sick" sense of
humor. It's a family thing.

The trip to the airport with Clay and his friends as they embarked on
their adventure on the West Coast can only be categorized as a "classic

moment" in life. The scene at the airport: Clay and his friend (who had his nipple pierced and a gold earring in it. Try to ignore that!); Clay's friend-girl who sported a head of hair frizzed out about a foot which resulted from a wild ride in a convertible to the airport; and gay friends..deliberately and most obviously gay, who were dressed outrageously, prissy-walking (my term) and giggling. Bringing up the tail end of this procession were the "straight" people: my single girlfriend, 12-year old daughter and one of her more open-minded girlfriends and me, the confused, distraught, but smiling, mother. Now that I look back, I think everyone was high except me, the younger kids, and my friend. Even we had been happily sipping Bloody Marys all afternoon.

I cannot say that being around openly hugging and kissing people of the same sex for the first time, and then going into the public arena with them was exactly fun, but it was an **EXPERIENCE.** Adding to this emotionally-charged atmosphere was the sadness I was feeling at watching Clay leaping out of my reach and my life and into a strange new world I would never know. It was my sincere hope that this man who claimed to love Clay would be sweet and protective of him and bring him some measure of happiness and satisfaction. This was the same hope I have always had for each of my children, for all my family, and for me. I remember asking this man to take good care of my baby. Little did we know about the "good life" in California.

In 1982 I took the plunge again and married a sweet, charming alcoholic against the pleadings of my daughter. We bought a really nice home, had some good friends, and life seemed pretty good. During the following two years my third son entered college, married, had a child, and divorced. I began to suspect the family might not be operating on all our cylinders. We definitely were not playing the game of life in a healthy manner.

In 1984 I began a job which was rewarding and enjoyable, we were comfortable in our new home and our "family" status. I was beginning to think that life was getting more stable, and that I could be married to this man for 50 years. He drank, but was sociable and likable and had a wonderful, loving family who made me feel important and accomplished. And, then..bingo.. my husband was transferred to another city during my daughter's senior year in high school. My interpretation of this move was that his alcohol problem was affecting his job, and they liked him so much, they moved him to protect him. The move seriously affected my daughter and deprived her of the joy of spending her last year of high school with all her friends. She tried to stay in our hometown. The plan was for her brothers to watch over her until she graduated. This plan did not work.

They all lived in one apartment complex, and the boys were busy with their own lives. She was not in a protected environment. She learned to party on a higher(?) plain, but realized she was out of her league.

Annie felt that her brothers not only expected her to carry her own load, but to pick up after them and babysit. She was used to "Mama" and felt so alone that one day she tearfully called and said she'd had enough of "independence" and wanted to be with me. This was a hard decision for an 18-year old.

We had moved to a town centered around the oil industry in another part of the state. I found a good job and made some friends who became my lifelong allies. My daughter also made lots of friends. They were from very rich families and had more elaborate party habits than she had encountered in our small eastern Oklahoma town. They were able to afford much more "sophisticated" drugs and played more "grown-up" games.

Okay, so now I was struggling with my growing inability to live with my husband's alcohol habit and the problems resulting from that habit, added to the mounting pressures of my children's struggles, plus coping with an energy- and time-consuming job. I just did not have the strength to cope with everything. The one part of my life I thought I could do something about was my marriage. I began distancing myself from the marriage and its demands on my energy, despite Al-Anons and a brief run at counseling. The old gut feeling that my "self" was being threatened was about to spur me to make another big move.

CLAY'S GOOD TIMES
—PRELUDE TO HELL

About this time, Clay began making some contact…a few inroads of communication…a phone call, a letter, a card…a glimpse into his life. Until then, I had only fleeting glimpses into Clay's life in Los Angeles and Long Beach. He was able to see the world, traveled to New York City, Washington, D.C., Canada, the Caribbean, made friends in all walks of life, walked on the "wild side"…enjoyed the best, suffered the worst. Clay fell in and out of love, had his heart broken, flirted and enjoyed being good looking and talented….just like many other human beings. He had a good work ethic and could make a home…but he loved to feel good. He loved to get high, to get drunk, to dull the pain….to really have fun.. to dance, sing and generally raise hell. I'm sure it was not always fun and games, but it was life as he chose it and it was full.

About that time, rumors of a strange malady affecting gay men in San Francisco. Ding! Warning bell! Ignore that. More calls. Two calls from the hospital "Mom, I have a lung infection and have been very ill." What I didn't know was that he was struggling with pneumocystis, and at that time, they were saying that two bouts with pneumocystis would be fatal. Then, the quiet but urgent call, "Mom, I have a new disease. We don't know a lot about it, but it's serious. You know I've been sick. I'm okay right now. But you need to find some help—a support group—here are some numbers to call. Don't worry."

I knew he was in trouble. My panicky mother's heart told me to get to him and make everything all better. I was very frightened. Clay and I decided I should visit sunny California. Clay wanted to share some of the beauty in his life..the flowers, the ocean air, the beach, the openness of California, and to meet his dog, Annabelle. This was a chance to share some of Clay's life, meet his friends, understand more, touch my son again. I was so excited. California was beautiful; I had never seen the ocean. Clay's friends were sweet and thoughtful…and they were dying of this strange malady which had just been given an official name..Acquired Immuno Deficiency Syndrome..AIDS. Clay had survived bouts with pnuemocystis, shingles, was afflicted with thrush, herpes and mild Kaposi's Sarcoma. He had been working as a counselor and educator with AIDS patients in Los Angeles. He had a working knowledge of the system, the services available, and the medications being tested and those on the market which might be "the answer" to a longer life. He was prolonging his own life by asserting his powerful personality in ways which forced "the system" to put him on AZT before the "official" criteria was met for administering this new drug. Clay was able to stay active and alive much longer than the 18 months the medical profession was predicting until certain death, because of his knowledge of all aspects of the epidemic. He altered his lifestyle and activities and began his long struggle for life.

Let me share a letter Clay wrote to me from California after dropping the bomb about his condition. This little missal gives a pretty good description of the life he was living at that time.

August 25, 1987

Dear Mom,

Ha! You thought it would never happen. I actually meant to write Friday, but, ooops, my energy went down to zero and took a nap instead. (I'd better write smaller, I can't afford stationery).

It's another ho-hum 72.4 º day and I'm anxiously awaiting the god-damned mailperson who is carrying my disability check which, *if* received in time, will cover the flotilla of rubber checks I wrote this weekend. One of these days, I will learn that the "rule of 13's" states that any moneys owed you will come one day later for any check writ-ten in anticipation of receiving them.

I've been a little "blah" this weekend, though certainly not through lack of activity. Saturday the …(Community Center) had its annual Great Gatsby Fundraiser. I wore a grey pinstripe tux with tails and braided my ponytail into a hop-sing. (Here he drew me a picture) Sunday we had a PWA (translation: Persons with AIDS)social at Steve Klar's house. All this activity is neat-o but sometimes I'd really like to do *nothing*. It seems as though sometimes we forget we *really are* sick.

I'm training a replacement at work. He, of course, is trying to be all things to all people and has not learned the limitations or the capabili-ties of a caseworker. This is why we do "practicum". In about 12 weeks he won't be so green.

I was deeply saddened by the new of Rhonda's (his step-sister's daughter)child's death. After a while I get a sedimentation of grief and the dam just bursts. It reminds me of that horrible polyphonic song we sang in high school: "In Media Vita, …." (In the midst of life, we grieve)

I heard a recent saying at a meeting, though, which emphasized the positive side of the Life-Struggle. It regarded the tiny bonsai tree which embodies the philosophy "That which struggles most for life is the most beautiful."*

Anyway, I've got to go. Thanks for being there when I need to talk and also for all the love and support you've all given me. You are always in my thoughts and prayers.

Love,
Clay

*(A friend of mine in Ponca City, Oklahoma, Stacy Merrifield, created a picture of a gnarled bonsai tree with this saying on it when she heard about Clay. This picture hangs in my home to remind me of the beauty of those who struggle most for life. Thanks, Stacy.)

At this point, I was forced to acknowledge the lifestyle Clay had been leading. My real baptism of fire was when I read *And The Band Played On* by Randy Schiltz. I found out things I did not want to know about gay life, the developing specter called AIDS, and the government's hideous non-response to the growing epidemic. While I was visiting him, Clay shared parts of his life with me. He was a recovering alcoholic and narcotics addict. He had done it all and tried it all! He had traveled and met famous people…he had really had fun. I shared his hurts and triumphs for a brief moment. We tried to resolve the bitterness and differences, and I cherished the moments, hoping against hope that this wonderful, tender young man was not going to be taken.

I viewed the horror of these beautiful, educated, responsible men going to early, ugly deaths..ignored by their families, vilified by society, crucified by the government. Hell was here! One of the most dramatic moments was attending an AA meeting for gay men who all had AIDS. It was here that I felt the first real, all encompassing love I had ever experienced. I was surrounded by loving, caring precious individuals—doomed to death—but opening their arms and hearts to me. Some needed a mother's validation because they could never receive their own mother's acceptance..even as they walked into the arms of death. How could I pass the message on? Love and accept them now, because soon they'll be gone, and you will have missed it! You will have missed the life of the precious little human being you brought into the world 26 years ago! What does it matter that they don't love and make love in the manner society says they should? What difference will it make when they are gone?

Because of the fatigue which working full time can cause and the escalation of HIV symptoms when a person is tired, Clay had "retired" from a job he had held for nearly 5 years at an expensive restaurant in Los Angeles. He helped found Project Ahead, an entity to help those people suffering with AIDS avail themselves of all that was available in the system…to be their advocates. He was also instrumental in founding Being Alive, a support group whose purpose was to try to help people with AIDS live triumphantly and fully until the bitter end.

He sadly left California in 1988, leaving those dying friends and sunny, open beautiful California to come back to the place from which he had "escaped" seven years earlier. What a blow to his independence! What a hard pill to swallow at 28 years of age. Going home to be near someone who would care for him during his last years. He did not want to be alone, but it was a bitter pill to swallow. It was good that he came back to share himself with us. We were about to be sucked into the vortex of Hurricane Clay once more… but this time, we were linked by a virus.

BACK HOME AGAIN

Clay and I joined forces in October of 1988 in Oklahoma City wistfully hopeful that life would be good and we all could get to know each other again. I found a wonderful, beautiful old home to rent. And one bright and clear autumn day Clay drove a U-Haul truck over the mountains with his dog Annabelle and came back to me. This was two years after his diagnosis with full blown AIDS, and I was determined to do the "mother" thing. I didn't realize he was doing the "son" thing and was ready to take care of me and help me learn to be happy. I decided I would "take care" of him and braced myself for the worst, prepared to care for a sick son and that time was short. Thank God Clay had taken responsibility for his own life. He controlled his diet, his lifestyle, his thoughts, his medications..and except for several scary bouts with symptoms , was termed a "long term survivor"."

Clay was brown and smiling and looking healthy and fit when he bounded out of that truck with Annabelle. He loved that patrician looking house; his beautiful things would just fit in there. To make things even better, the house was in a "yuppy" neighborhood. He was such a snob..he had class. He was optimistic and fully aware of my fear of being able to make it financially. He reassured me that we would make it, because he had finally been certified for Social Security Disability and Medicaid. I had good work skills and worked the temps for a while and finally landed a job with a community newspaper. The paper and my boss were notoriously Republican and very right wing. This gave my

kids and friends a chuckle…a bleeding heart liberal in the midst of a den of Republicans. I learned a lot during those months. I was exposed to some very conservative Republicans who were very open about homosexuals and their getting their "just desserts". I could not keep quiet after reading one of our Oklahoma legislator's comments in a newspaper in Oklahoma City. Here's a portion of the letter I wrote: (I will leave this former Oklahoma state representative's name out)
"Dear ,

I am writing you with a sad and weary heart after reading your reply to Jerry West and Christopher S. Clason of OKC's Pride Network.

I object to your quoting scriptures out of context and of your statement that "Christ and God" speak to us regarding homosexuality. Carefully research your scriptures, Mr. _____. Find and send to me any place that Jesus referred to the sin of homosexuality. Jesus's primary message was for compassion, forgiveness, and love. He forgave those he touched—the lepers, the woman at the well—he didn't ask them how they got they go the disease. His best friends were sinners; he did not waste his precious time and message sitting with the church members of his time. He was not afraid to touch those who were rejected by society. *They* were his ministry………………

…My god is not punishing my son by "giving" him AIDs, any more than God is punishing people with lung cancer for smoking—does that make smoking a sin… an abomination?

Please do not include my gay son in the same category as child molesters and abusers, thieves, and arsonists. He and his friends are none of those—they work, worship, pay taxes, care for the sick and poor. They vote; they are the foundation of our philharmonic, ballet, drama—they are not hypocrites. They do fight back—fighting bigotry and ignorance.

…If I were the gays, I wouldn't have invited you to the parade. You do not represent the majority, thankfully, and you make me ashamed to be called a "heterosexual"."

I was angry at the world, at the injustice, at the disease.

Clay and I went on outings, listened to beautiful music, worked in the yard…and argued. It was a lot of work for both of us to give up our single lifestyles. The house did not have a washer and dryer, and dirty clothes became a bone of contention. Clay was teaching me that living with someone with AIDS entailed a lot of cleaning and care. One fact was clear by that time in the epidemic: HIV was transmissible through fluids. We kept bleach around for spills and cleaning. Clay admonished me not to use his toothbrush or razor, not to touch body fluids with bare hands. Of course, these are simple rules of hygiene good for all households.

We became part of a community stricken with AIDS. Clay knew how to seek out groups for support. We found sharing groups for families, for gays, for those interested in helping. These groups were full of health care workers and individuals dedicated to contributing love and support. We were all seeking all the information we could on this epidemic. Speculation and investigation brought new information every day, and with each new piece of information, hope that this new discovery would be the one which would cure the disease. For the present, we had to look for those ways which would stem off the inevitable onslaught of the virus's overtaking the immune system.

Those affected with HIV listened and absorbed methods others had devised for maintaining their dignity and retaining as good a quality of life as possible under the almost impossible circumstances. The disease itself was devastating, but the social and political death were just as vicious..maybe more so. What a load to carry. Discrimination and fear from all sides: work, friends, family..the whole nation..added to impending death. Support groups with lots of love and touching were our lifelines. The old life, the old friends, faded in the harsh light of dealing with the stigma of AIDS.

The news media were full of stories of militant groups demanding that the government be made accountable for its part in hiding the epidemic because of the overwhelming cases in the gay communities. No government agencies would admit that the alarming statistics which were a real threat to the whole nation..indeed, the whole world..had been pushed under the rug in hopes that it might control the homosexual movement and perhaps be an easy way to eliminate the problem of open homosexuality. In this case, the morality of those in control of the funding for research in our nation's capitol have dealt a hand of death to millions by lying about how the "millions for research" was being allocated. Those people who were involved in the government's decision to withhold funds and information about HIV, knowing that HIV was communicable and deadly, can take a lot of credit for the staggering numbers of those infected all over the world. Whom were they protecting?

In California, Texas , Florida and New York, not only support groups for the dying like Shanti emerged, but members of the health care community began to get organized to do the job the government should have been spearheading. They petitioned state and local governments to develop a curriculum for teaching the prevention of HIV. They began to form HIV clinics for testing , education, and prevention. The numbers of new infections was growing and the public began to ask what was being done to stop it..what was this thing called AIDS? The general community began to realize the enormity of the consequences of the epidemic and its effect on the world. All of a sudden, the world was losing a whole generation of young people: people in the arts, attorneys, world leaders, athletes, entertainers. These dead people were their neighbors, their pastors, their favorite movie stars. What was happening?

I must say that while the realities of the infection itself were being discovered, the horror of the social stigma began to rear its ugly head. The venom heaped upon those afflicted with HIV and their families is unforgivable and negates our nation's claim to being founded upon the premises of belief in God, and freedom to pursue life , liberty and happiness. It became all too clear to me that our beloved America had more serious problems than the budget and foreign policy. Every effort to educate the public met with great opposition from the so-called moral majority and those politicians who feared their power. Educating the country in the prevention of a disease spread by blood, semen and vaginal fluids would seem that the government was condoning sex outside of marriage. If the messages to save lives were too graphic, those hearing the message might get ideas and engage in activities they might not have thought about. Therefore those trying to educate were rendered ineffective by making the very subjects which must be addressed unacceptable or were completely eliminated.

A few militant groups, like Act Up, have managed to get some action on every front by making people angry. I am familiar with ACT UP because Clay was a part of these brave, informed young people who pushed people's faces in the facts. Some of their tactics were a little overboard, but it takes a pretty mean slap in the face to get the public's attention.

Countless groups of people, organized and individually, petitioned their congressmen and senators for funding for education, for funding for survival for those whose livelihood had been stripped from them by society and the disease, for funding for health care facilities, for nurseries for the surviving children of people who had died of AIDS, for anything showing that our government recognized the tremendous problem facing the nation and the world.

This was the "new world" Clay and AIDS brought me, and I will never be the same. If it had not been for the love and support of a group of mothers during those months of discovering the world of AIDS, I think our lives would have been unbearable. Clay and I were introduced to an AIDS Support and Education Group, which was functioning on a combination federal and state grant in Oklahoma City. Clay was very interested in working with this group as a caseworker, since he had gained so much experience in this field in Los Angeles. "The Plan", although undefined, would be for Clay to work through the state's health department on a program which was set up to coordinate the needs with the availability of services and funding. This income augmented by his Social Security disability income combined with the income I could bring in from working would allow us to live comfortably, although limited. I did not reckon with the politics and the intrigue and manipulation which are always a part of such programs. Clay had already dealt with this system in California, and was not too surprised when the promised job offer fell apart. He did not have the energy or time to play these political games again. As soon as the signs of the same problems began to emerge, Clay disengaged and began to look for alternatives.

I was appalled that the AIDS issue needed to be addressed and the need was so great, but the criteria for hiring help was so encumbered by bureaucratic red tape. The programs were strangled by that red tape, and have operated on a roller coaster for the past 10 years. A lot of good has been done and many programs have emerged from these beginnings, but many dying people and their families have not been given the help, information and services they needed at that specific time. They..including Clay..did not have the luxury of time to work through egos, ignorance and bigotry to have a program implemented and funded. This continues.

Clay was a spokesman from the beginning. Not only was he member of ACT UP, but a contributing member to the media. He was a favorite for interviews on the Oklahoma City television stations. He knew his facts, he was articulate, polite and handsome, and he pulled no punches. He wrote countless letters to politicians, newspaper editors, magazines, religious officials and anyone else he thought could aid in getting the information out to the public and in getting funding to research HIV/AIDS and help in treating and caring for those already afflicted.

Clay had learned over the years to create a home filled with beautiful paintings, vases, flowers, and ringing with beautiful music, on a budget. I had acquired some experience with budgeting myself, so despite our limited income, our days were full and poignantly sweet. He decided I needed a dog of my own, since he had a dog and a cat, so he brought home from a support meeting a precious salt and pepper miniature Schnauzer at Christmas for me. He named my new little companion Alexander Beauregard. This dog was affectionately known as Alex to the kids, but he was always little Alexander to me.

Over the next few years Alexander became my companion and confidante, just as Clay's black and white Springer Spaniel ,Annabelle, was his connection to staying alive. Clay's animals were the only living things who gave him unconditional love, loyalty, and respect. Clay returned that love by taking good care of them, lavishing them with care and discipline. When he was the sickest, Clay worried more about his dogs than he did himself, and spent many hours teaching the family and his friends how to care for his beloveds.

Clay's father visited with us in Oklahoma City. This visit gave Clay an expectation that his father cared for him and was at last accepting him. That same fall, my sister and her husband, who are strong born again Christians, came by to visit. Contacts with these family members bolstered our supply of hope, which was in short supply. We were so isolated from any semblance of a family. We conjured up a hope .. a hope time would show to be false . That hope was that our family loved us once again, and would be there for us during these times of trouble and worry. This hope did not come to fruition.

Clay had rejoined the Catholic Church, only to switch to Judaism (which he had embraced when he was a teenager) once again. I am sure that a lot of this decision to change was brought about by the Catholic Church's stand on abortion and homosexuals. He thoroughly embraced orthodox Judaism, studying Hebrew and kibitzing with the members of the synagogue..who seemed to have cared less if he was gay or not. He always amazed people with the knowledge he had of religions, languages, countries, civilizations. Clay had been blessed with a remarkable genius, a photographic memory, and an insatiable curiosity. He was a student of life, and later became a teacher of life to all of us.

In September of 1989 Clay decided he wanted to live in a bigger house and Annie, my daughter, could live with us to help with expenses…and we could have a washer and dryer. We would be one big happy family. Wrong! This arrangement lasted only 4 months, and Clay decided he felt well enough to live alone…he was wanting to date again…and he was going to continue his education at the Central State University in Edmond, a suburb of Oklahoma City. Let me tell you…his decisions were always absolute and this one made life very hard for my daughter and me.

So, my daughter, Clay and I began living on "our own" again. Clay became increasingly involved in the activist arena and was a constant guest on Oklahoma City news programs. He attended AIDS conferences in Washington, D.C., and began swimming on a gay swimming team. He and some friends participated in the Gay Olympics in Canada. Clay was an excellent swimmer and carried some medals back to the U.S. from those Olympics. Clay and his friends were active in the arts, along with their activist activities, but much of his time was spent ministering to those suffering and dying.

At that time, in early 1990's, people with AIDS and those who knew they were infected with HIV spent most of their waking moments searching for the most effective mix of medical care and medications. Access to this care and medications involved a lot of investigation and sometimes, sadly, politics. God help you if you made one of the coordinators of a support group or a member of the limited medical profession an enemy. You might need them when the chips are down. Clay became very active with the Pro-Choice movement. He was an advocate of women's rights. He was an advocate of animal rights. He was an advocate of children's rights. He was a defender of those who were on the outside. Clay was making his mark on the world while he had time and strength.

Clay enrolled in Central State University for two semesters. The next year, he transferred to Oklahoma University and moved to Norman. He carried a full load of classes with the goal of graduating. Dying was out of his vocabulary. He wanted life, and he wanted to learn more about life. He loved learning and carried a 4.0 average in Spanish, anthropology, Hebrew, and classes I cannot even pronounce. I was amazed to find his report cards and congratulatory letters advising him that he was on the Dean's list or the President's list…every single semester.

Clay became one of the Oklahoma University campus newspaper *The Oklahoma Daily's* controversial columnists during 1990 and 1991. Able to express himself verbally and on paper, Clay used this little column as a forum for his philosophies, experiences and opinions. He didn't pull any punches, but managed to present some good arguments and ideas. I would call them "thought provoking" and probably provoked more than thoughts when people read them. These articles expressed a lot of anger in some of the columns, but definitely presented the facts according to Clay. Here are some excerpts from his 1991 contributions. And they do not necessarily express my own personal opinion.

June 12, 1991

"Fear, loathing and the great AIDS betrayal

Millions of Americans gathered this past weekend to welcome home our troops and to congratulate them on a job well-done.

While middle America wallowed in the mud of its newly found national pride, I watched aghast (if only for 20 minutes) this orgy of self-congratulation and military hardware put on by the big pink men in blue suits.

Yup, we whooped their Iraqui asses. We showed that pesky Sadam Hussein an attack on a sovereign state would not be tolerated—by slaughtering more than 100,000 of his countrymen.

The only ways I can describe my thoughts while viewing this welcoming-home spectacle are with the words *alienation* and *disgust.*

I do not understand why people get excited while viewing "smart" weapons, which are designed to kill as many people from a great distance as possible. I do not understand the national adulation doled out for that Care-Bear-with-an-Uzi, General Norman Schwarzkopf.

Most of all, I cannot comprehend why it takes the near-annihilation of a vastly outgunned country to muster the national resolve of this nation.

110,000 Americans have died of AIDS to date. The stories of many of these people are the stories of heroes who have fought both a debilitating disease and the hysteria produced by ignorance.

AIDS has produced a new breed of "patient," one that is fundamentally involved in the improvement of his own health and health care, as well as the improvement of the lot of others affected by the disease.

Media attention to people with AIDS is usually sketchy, and often focuses upon "innocent" people who were infected through blood products. These reports largely reinforce the ignorance they *claim* to seek to dispel, that people deserve this illness.

We certainly do not see Linda Cavanaugh, the local dominatrix of TV-land kitsch, gushing nightly about the plight of people with AIDS in the face of an unresponsive government and health care establishment.

Instead we are treated nightly to monosyllabic editorials disguised as news that sing the praises of men with medals and patriot missiles.

George Bush mustered up a bucket of alligator tears when he spoke of those 300-or-so who died during Operations Desert Shield and Storm.

But the only emotion I ever detect when our Commander-in-chief speaks of AIDS is a cynical assurance that the government is doing enough to curb the epidemic of HIV, which has been far more costly to America than any diabolical plot Saddam Hussein could hatch.

The most dramatic response the Bush clan has generated in response to AIDS has been to place a melancholy candle in a solitary White House window on World AIDS Day. Thanks, Babs, for the token gesture, but an annual candle doesn't take the place of any *sincere* commitment to battle AIDS.

The real attitude of George toward the HIV epidemic is reflected in his appointment of a reactionary Surgeon General Antonio Novello, who has quietly unraveled the policies of C. Everett Koop and replaced them with the anti-sexual and unrealistic policy of *Just Say No.*

George's opposition to the inclusion of AIDS as a protected disability in the Americans With Disabilities Act tells the true tale o his administration's AIDS policy.

The message to me is clear: *take cover, because it's open season on you.*

I have a genuine feeling my government has betrayed me, so excuse me if I don't gush with patriotic pride when I hear the national anthem, or fret when George's ticker sputters occasionally. Any lump in my throat that results from seeing Old Gory pass by can be quickly resolved with a spoon or syrup of ipecac.

Clay Shear is a Norman senior majoring in Spanish/anthropology. ".
June 20, 1991

"Don't blame the individual for having AIDS

I have spoken about living AIDS and the problems presented by the HIV epidemic to an array of individuals and groups. One topic invariably comes up: SEX.

Without fail, at least one individual asks if I still have sex. When I answer with an enthusiastic "yes", one or more individuals asks if I'm careful not to infect others. The answer to this questions is also yes, but its condescending and patronizing message bears additional response.

First of all, there aren't *others.* I only have one sexual partner and we are in a mutually monogamous, loving and lifelong relationship.

The message implied in the word *others* is that people with HIV infection are non-stop and insatiable sex machines, like characters from "Barbarella". This is a lie brought to you by the same people who call mosquitoes "flying hypodermic syringes".

The more serious implication contained in the words *"are you being careful?"* is that people with HIV infection are morally irresponsible and regularly traipse about the sexual highways and byways of life infecting unwary virgin Republicans.

While I admit such a prospect is titillating, reliable studies and personal experience demonstrate that individuals who *know* they are HIV infected take great pains to protect others from infection.

But people with HIV infection are not the only players in this game. Every individual who is sexually active, and I confidently assume that *everyone* is, bears the *personal responsibility to* protect him or herself from HIV infection.

Barring sexual coercion, *blame* does not exist in the realm of HIV infection, but *responsibility* does. The difference between blame and responsibility is simple: blame is an abdication of responsibility.

Blame is a practice that segregates our population into us and them, those who are innocent and those who are guilty, the deserving and the undeserving. Unfortunately, this practice has molded our nation's and our government's policies toward AIDS.

As recently as 1990, the United States Congress debated a measure which criminalized the donation of blood by people who knew they were HIV-infected.

Does anyone *really* believe that people who are HIV-infected line up outside donation centers, just *itching* to have an 18-gauge needle rammed into their veins?

State legislatures rushed to pass laws that made it a crime to infect others with HIV. The Oklahoma Legislature, always a bastion of principle and morality, passed a law which made it a crime to *intend* to cause another person to become infected with HIV. The innocent white folks had to be protected from an invisible horde of contagious, recalcitrant perverts.

These laws are example of a solution in desperate need of a problem. Only a handful of cases has been successfully prosecuted and could have been adequately handled with existing public and reckless endangerment laws, but American lawmakers had to jump on the blame-the-buggers bandwagon.

The pro-active approach of personal responsibility has made dramatic progress in curb in the transmission of HIV among Gay men in San Francisco, New York, and Los Angeles.

The seroconversion rate, the number of persons testing positive for HIV who previously tested negative, is near zero among Gay men in San Francisco, and can be largely attributed to massive and explicit educational efforts.

This is solid evidence that HIV-infected individuals, when given accurate information on how to prevent the infection of others with HIV, behave responsibly. It also shows that, by teaching every individual to take immediate responsibility for his or her own health, the epidemic can be brought into check.

Sex *is*. It is an integral component of human individuals and societies. It is an integral component of my life. Blaming sex, or individuals who have sex, or people who donate blood, will not prevent AIDS. Education and an attack on ignorance will."

I am glad that we have this written record of Clay's views, however biased they may seem. These words provide a written testament of the history of the AIDS epidemic and how individuals who are HIV-infected are affected by politics and prejudice. Of course, most of these words are calculated to elicit *response and action*.

While trying to educate the world around him about the epidemic and being gay in the USA, Clay managed to maintain his superior scholastic record while working at the Hillel Foundation, keeping house, taking care of his animals, himself, and his friends. He had moved into a house with his companion, Harold, and Harold's dog,

Howard, and with various cats. And he and Harold committed themselves to each and exchanged rings to signify that commitment.

From 1989 through the fall of 1991, I like to think Clay lived a full
life…hiking and camping in the Arbuckles south of Oklahoma City,
collecting rocks, taking pictures, riding his mountain bike, competitive
swimming in both school and gay meets, and cooking. He liked
Norman. Norman's bohemian atmosphere fit Clay's open style of living
and thinking. However, he became so involved in life again, he began
engaging in using drugs and began drinking again. At the same time, he
was having increasingly more frequent bouts with advanced symptoms
of AIDS. Because of the pain of the Kaposi's lesions and resulting
chemotherapy, some lung problems and the constant battle with
depression and fear, he was on some pretty powerful barbiturates. Some
of his friends began not only to take advantage of his hospitality, but
began to help themselves to his drugs. His life was becoming a jumble
again.

I had moved to the Austin area and back to my "native" Texas, after
my father died in March of 1991, thinking that maybe if Clay got sicker,
we could live in Daddy's house there by the lake. I did not realize that
my sister and her family (and all of my family) did not want Clay to
come to that house because they were fearful that he would leave germs
on the toilet, and one of them would get "it". They did not even want to
be near Clay…not only because of the disease…but because they
believed him to be the vilest of sinners. Clay and I visited with my
mother and my brother and his father's mother in Fort Worth one
Sunday. This visit was very painful. I am sure this scenario has been
repeated in many families over the past 15 years. My family members
were polite and friendly, but they were terrified and fearful. They did
not want Clay to touch them and practically ran when Clay would get
near. He needed a hug, to be touched, to be reassured that he had a family. His father's family members were more realistic, compassionate and
helpful in many ways. After that visit, Clay and I knew they were

relieved when we left. It was obvious that they did not want us around, nor did they want to know anything about the disease or how it was affecting our lives.

I had visited with Clay in Norman several times and noted the people who were in his life. Some were really good friends who shared their lives with him…even let him be at the birth of their baby…and some were leaches.

In about October of 1992, I decided to drive through Norman on my way to visit friends, having moved back to Oklahoma in January. I had missed those hills and people so much that I found a job with the March of Dimes and moved into a little apartment in Muskogee, and eventually went to work in Tahlequah, my favorite town in the world. When I walked on to Clay's porch, I was horrified at the disarray, and how overwhelmed he was with the everyday duties of keeping house, caring for himself…and picking up after the others. He was too weak and sick to be doing those things..it was just too much. I remember that day so vividly. I looked into Clay's big, blue eyes and said, "Honey, this is it. We knew this time would come. Are you ready to come home to Tahlequah with me where we will be safe? I have friends and a support system and my job and can be near you." It was a tragic, tender moment, but Clay was visibly relieved that he wouldn't have to carry all of the responsibility anymore.

I quickly went back to Tahlequah and found a house out in the country..not the best in the world..but a place where Clay could have his three dogs and cat!! He would not give any of them up, even though persons with compromised immune systems are not supposed to have a lot of pets around…especially cats and birds. This house, too, was in the middle of a field with cattle in them, with only a barbed wire fence around the house to keep the cattle out…but wouldn't keep the dogs in. Another challenge…I learned how to hook chicken wire to barbed wire around about a half-acre lot…in the cold and wind. But I did it!

We moved on a cold, drizzly day. When we arrived in Norman at the house, nothing had been done. No one had helped Clay get things together. Clay had rented a U-Haul truck and my son, his daughter, and my daughter were there to pack up. We felt helpless...the task seemed overwhelming. After a few calls and with the help of a few of his real friends (God bless 'em) we not only packed up, but gathered up, cleaned up, and wrestled all of Clay's books, tools, and worldly goods into our cars and the truck! It was a horrible experience, but we landed in our own little home in Tahlequah late that night.

THE BEGINNING
OF THE END

Clay enjoyed the beauty of the location of that house. He could look out the windows and watch the birds and animals and could use his "green thumb" to grow a profusion of flowers. And he could use the expensive camera he bought to make photographic memories of the sights he enjoyed. He decorated that beat-up old farmhouse with beautiful "cha chas" as he called them. He brought his talent for planting a yard full of lush grass and overflowing flower beds to our new home. My new friends in the Green Country AIDS Coalition became our support. They would come to help around the house. The took Clay for long drives in the countryside…to wade in the spring-fed creeks, and hike over the hills discovering wild flowers and rock formations.

I kept my apartment in Muskogee…for my own sanity. This was a private place I could go to scream and grieve. I had read the book *The Screaming Room, A Mothers Journal of Her Son's Struggle* by Barbara Peabody, suggested by some knowing friends and was beginning to get an inkling what that mother went through. I had a haven where I could be quiet and visit with my friends. I know Clay did not understand why I kept that apartment.

He thought it was an unnecessary expense, but it was my connection to reality, to my own identity, to escape the nightmare. Poor Clay…he could not escape the nightmare. He did not ask for sympathy and he remained in control. He lived with dignity, and tried to help as much as possible with the daily routine of working and living. His daily routine consisted of maintaining his strength and managing his pain. Much of his time was spent wrestling with the maze of problems involved in the complications of the paperwork involved in filing claims with Medicaid and Social Security and working within the system set up to administer those programs.

People struggling with the disease and its ramifications must also deal with the social services system. The difficult development of an accessible service system for people with HIV and AIDS paralleled the time line that Clay was walking with the disease. There were times when Clay encountered workers involved in the federal and state Departments of Health who either refused to work with gay people with the disease or treated their prospective clients with less than a professional, helping attitude. This type of behavior and treatment abated after a time, but those who manifested this attitude with Clay found themselves either out of a job or called on the carpet. Clay gave them no quarter. He and I both felt that those people whose vocation is to serve should be educated and trained to be able to handle those in need…no matter what the disability or the cause of it. Moral judgements have no place in the services field. In private, a person can have his own prejudices, but not in this particular workplace.

Clay was not only fatigued from the illness but suffering battle fatigue from fighting the system. Being introduced to the gentleness and openness of Cherokee County's health care workers and social service personnel was a breath of fresh air for Clay and me. They were willing to help and depended on Clay to share his experience with the system, so that they could be of more service. Many doctors in rural areas are willing to treat those people with HIV and AIDS, but they lack the experience, training and facilities to effectively and aggressively treat the disease. Initially, family physicians want to protect the families from the diagnosis of HIV and from the social isolation and sometimes violent community reaction to that diagnosis. And, I suppose, often they do not recognize that this could be HIV, because they have known the person since childhood and may be unaware of a lifestyle which would put the patient at risk. And, often, they just treat the symptoms as they crop up…allowing HIV to progress at an accelerated rate. These patients can have a risk of dying faster.

Fortunately, Clay was able to contact his physician in Oklahoma City for a referral to a doctor in Tulsa, which is just about 60 miles from Tahlequah, when he developed a rare lung virus and his Kaposi's lesions began to increase on his body. It takes a special type of physician and support personnel to treat HIV and AIDS. These offices face an overwhelming task of keeping up with the new medications and balancing treatments for the enormously complicated symptoms, plus managing the paperwork for claims. They are fighting a ticking time bomb in every patient. They have taken on the terrible responsibility of trying to match the most effective treatment with the patient's lifestyle and the patient's finances. They are in the difficult position of not only providing medical care, but psychological support and counseling….for those looking at certain death. Since Clay's death in 1994, medications and treatments have been developed which prolong life and improve the quality of that life. The social aspect has improved somewhat and the country has become more aware of the impact of HIV and AIDS as more and more people become acquainted with the disease when family members or friends become ill.

In 1992 and 1993, when Clay was experiencing multiple symptoms and complications, the few doctors in the big cities in Oklahoma were overwhelmed, and probably still are. The hospitals were still not set up to care for the multiple problems people with AIDS experience. I suspect they still are not.

It is hard for me to believe some of the experiences Clay and I had in dealing with the prejudices and fears. It is almost unbelievable that the worst experiences were within the very systems sworn to uphold the sanctity of preserving life in the name of the Church. For example, during the summer of 1992, Clay felt that he should visit his grandmother who was in the hospital in Fort Worth. I agreed to pick him up in Norman, then we decided to take a trip to our "lake place" to hang out and enjoy some of the uniqueness of the Hill Country of Texas, after that visit to Fort Worth.

I'll explain our "lake place", and then get back to the experience of 1992 in Fort Worth. After my father died in 1991 in the Austin-area of Texas on Lake Travis, he left his home and estate to my sister and me, his only children. Since I was single and Clay was better and getting along pretty well in Oklahoma, my sister and I thought I could move into the house,clean it up, and make some improvements so the families could use it for get-togethers. I could look for a job and have a "new life". My own purpose also included a plan that Clay could come live with me in that peaceful spot when the time came, and we could have a peaceful life and still be near the Austin area. Austin seemed to be pretty progressive and accepting of gays and the whole AIDS epidemic since it was and still is an university-oriented atmosphere. And the climate allowed for relaxed living. The acre of land Daddy owned was in a lakefront community in what Texans call "the Balcones"…rugged hills of limestone and cedars..and wonderful clear lakes. The house was built for a weekend retreat for a couple, and he had bought it when he was in his 70's and converted it to his hermit's retreat. He furnished it in the manner most single people do…as simply as possible. Half of the house was used as the repository for his multitude of radio equipment. Daddy had been a U. S. Marine radioman in the eastern theatre during World War II, and had continued in that field as he tried to assimilate back into society in the late 40's. During the 50's, he migrated to central Texas and began his career as a Navy MARS radio operator. He was one of those special people who contacted families for those young people on their first ventures into the world of "keeping the peace"..or as we have known several times: "war". He was there to pass on Christmas and birthday greetings to families and to service men and women who were hungry to make contact. Daddy sat many hours in his radio lair during emergency situations and received many awards for his dedication and help. David Baker—call letters WA5QVP—was a respected member of the short wave radio community..and known all over the world.

Now Daddy was an eccentric, too, so Clay and the rest of the "black sheep" of our family have come by it "honest". He was super intelligent and unable to cope with people as a whole. An artist, an avid reader, interested in learning, a music lover. And a recluse.

Anyway, after he died, I moved in, hopefully, as I said, for a new beginning for me and maybe a happier ending for Clay's life. I did not reckon with unforgiving judgement against Clay's lifestyle and fear of the disease he might spread to my sister's family. I'm not sure if they were more fearful of the homosexuality or the "germs". Since my sister and I were to share the house, and they were to be able to come spend time at the lake, they did not want Clay there at all. They were afraid that he would leave a germ on the toilet, or that the virus was air borne. No matter what the medical studies were proving; no matter that I was her sister and needed love and protection..and my child needed love and understanding. They wanted me out. The faith community they are so wrapped up in…and I certainly respect their faithfulness and beliefs..seems to have some convoluted idea that the AIDS crisis is a government cover-up and that all of the facts about how the disease is spread have been hidden from the public. I've never figured that out…for what purpose would the "government" lie about the epidemic?

I had been there for just a few months, but realized that this arrangement was not going to work. I honestly had not understood that they thought I was only going to be there for a little while , find a job in Austin, and move out, leaving the house for just vacations. This plan did not include Clay.

Nevertheless, my kids and I really did enjoy "Baker's Acres" during those months. Thanksgiving of 1991 all of the kids, including Clay and his friend Harold, some of their friends ,and of course all of their dogs and my little dog Alexander, gathered for a gala holiday. We have this precious holiday on video. Not precious like traditional American Thanksgiving gatherings....this was a really combo Baker-Shear-Huddleston all-out Texas bash. Daddy's house has a wonderful patio and covered barbecue grill—perfect for outdoor gatherings. The weather was very warm and conditions were ripe for a celebration. The only ones missing were Matt and his daughter. Matt had graduated from optometry school and had joined the U.S. Army and was serving at Ft. Irwin, California, during Desert Storm.

After cooking lots of turkey and trimmings, and after lots of drinking and carrying on, we decided to have a Trivial Pursuit-O-Rama, on the patio in the middle of the night. Everyone was very mellow and full of food and "spirits" and Dan, the self appointed bartender, decided to prepare a large batch of Margarita's. To be hospitable, we invited the neighbors who had befriended Daddy during his years at the lake. Well, not just to be hospitable...two of the young neighbors are accomplished musicians and really congenial and fun. One neighbor, a Cajun-turned-Texan, was our "guest of honor" and came over to play with us for Thanksgiving. Dan was double dosing him with tequila, and I think we nearly killed him. He wandered off in the woods after midnight, never to be seen again that night. He quipped the next day that my kids "sho' know how to pah-ty".

The marathon Trivial Pursuit game continued way into the night...and it was a true battle. Clay, with his photographic memory, was nearly impossible to beat. But the group as a whole were all pretty smart and well read and well rounded, so the answers and reactions were an explosion of hilarity. I have never laughed so much. I just love my children and their many friends. The way they take life in both hands and LIVE IT. Clay's friends were no exception. Except they are all dead.

This memorable holiday, Clay was in his glory..he was with the man he loved, his brothers and sisters, friends, dogs, and Mom. We laughed and laughed and loved and loved. Precious moments…precious memories.

Soon after, I packed up my belonging and left Texas and my father's last home. I thought, "I don't need this rejection and cruelty. They can have the place." So I worked with my sister and her husband and sold my half to them. They now use it as a retreat for themselves and other Christian couples… a far cry from my little "heathen's haven".

We still loved Daddy's place, so the kids and I sought out the owner of a piece of property two lots away. Daddy had hired this man to help him get around, since he was weakened by a congestive heart condition and poor circulation, and had helped him buy this run-down house on stilts and paid for his septic system. Daddy wanted this little family to have a place to live, and he needed help desperately. A little before Daddy died, this man left Texas, and left the property empty. We searched for him and accidentally found him in the southeast, and purchased the property, paid off the delinquent taxes, and became joint landowners. This place is now our "retreat".

Clay did not get to have much interaction with my father because Daddy was very uncompromising and harsh on his grandchildren. He just did not know how to accept people as they were. He sure wasn't going to accept a queer, although they certainly would have enjoyed each other. They both had that intellectual curiosity and affinity for music, art and language which made them so alike. Oh, what we miss because we saddle our relationships with "conditions". Conditional love…what an oxymoron. So sad…so wasteful. Maybe my father and my son are sharing some of eternity together.

Back to the summer of 1992—Clay's wonderful Catholic grandmother was very ill with cancer at All Saints Hospital in Fort Worth. The boys and I had kept an open relationship with their father's family. I must say that this family was just the opposite of mine. When they found out that Clay was gay and had AIDS, they found out as much as they could about the disease, talked with their doctors, prayed about it, and opened their arms to him. They did not condone or condemn his lifestyle. His grandmother offered part of the funds she had set aside for her grandchildren. Clay felt so close to this grandmother and was very concerned about her condition. She was a devout and faithful Catholic and was, of course, in a Catholic hospital. Clay had a sweet and poignant visit with her. However, before we left for this trip, Clay had a medical condition on his thigh which required that it be removed. This incision was still healing and draining, which was not good for Clay or for those around him. I must emphasize again how aware Clay was that he should not endanger anyone around him. He took great precaution to be sure that he did not infect anyone else.

The doctors who had done the procedure in Oklahoma City had advised him to get the dressing changed within 24 hours. Clay was on Medicare and very knowledgeable about what needed to be done, had his paperwork with him regarding his condition and the wound, and he was in a lot of pain. Since we were in a hospital, we went down to the Emergency Room of this great Catholic hospital. They were cold and rude and refused to treat him. This was so embarrassing and frustrating. I could not believe it. Now I knew what these people had been experiencing. That hospital had been supported with the finances and prayers of this family for decades, and they could not live up to their Hippocratic oath and treat him. No wonder Clay embraced Judaism after that experience.

He had become hardened to reactions like this, but we were surprised that 7 years into the epidemic people were still reacting so inhumanely. I was devastated and grieved for my poor proud sick son. We found an emergency medical facility on I-35 on the way out of town who treated him gently and with dignity. While we were waiting there, I called my Mother and brother to meet us out there. They really were uncomfortable with Clay coming to the house, and I thought this might give them a chance to spend some time with him. It was an awkward visit, and I could see my mother and brother were a little shaken at our experience. I think it may have given them a little insight as to how ugly Clay's fight for survival could be.

STAYING ALIVE

While Clay was in Norman in 1992, the small purple dots on Clay's torso and legs began to grow into angry lesions. These painful skin cancers are called Kaposi's Sarcoma or K.S. and plague most people with HIV and AIDS. They are one of the signs of a seriously compromised immune system—a sign that the immune system is failing in its battle against disease and infections. Patients with K.S., whether they have AIDS or not, must undergo the same treatments that other cancer patients endure to try to control the cancer. Clay was undergoing chemotherapy treatment to contain the growth of these lesions. A few weeks before he moved to Tahlequah, he had been given powerful doses of radiation on his legs and his feet for the lesions. During the third round of the radiation , they had seriously burned him, and his feet and legs were painfully swollen from this radiation burn. He could hardly walk. The pain of the K.S. combined with the treatment required an increase in Clay's morphine prescription.

Pain management is a big problem for people like Clay, who have been hard core drug users. Clay had abused drugs. As he explained to a home health care nurse who was concerned that Clay could not give himself the daily injections of Interferon, he told her he had shot up in every vein and orifice in his body and was quite familiar with injections. Said lightly, but with a serious undertone…he knew he was paying the price for that type of knowledge.

During the last few months and weeks, we had to travel to Tulsa to the cancer treatment facility for chemotherapy, which had to be followed up with injections to counteract the nausea caused by chemotherapy. These were just added medications and treatments to the myriad of other prescriptions Clay was taking: Diflucan, an antifungal; Zovirax, AZT; Ddi, in conjunction with AZT; various drugs for depression and anxiety;

I cannot begin to describe the years, months, weeks, and days as the clock was ticking and the hidden disintegration of Clay's body was progressing. I can only describe and try to recover the great energy that Clay possessed—demanded—at times..and shared at other times. If I squint up my eyes and push my mind back and visualize the entire walk, I can see the thread of light and energy. Clay had tapped into that mystical field through his meditating and studying and had found his way to trapping—no—absorbing, maintaining, building that energy..so as to maintain LIFE. He absorbed and adsorbed through his interaction with the earth, music, art, animals, food, religions..even the rocks and flowers had interaction with Clay..and vice versa.

As his body lost ground, Clay's mind and spirit energized him. Now I understand why he could not be around most people..or a lot of people. They took his energy. There were days when I must have drained him, but there were times when he had to depend on my energy..I did not realize the dynamics at the time. He could rest and relate to Sara, his God-sent soulmate..our helper and friend. She rejuvenated him through quiet meditation, sharing walks and rides through the country, massages. I could tell when Clay had been with Sara..he was full of energy, warmth and well-being. God bless her..what would we have done without her!?

Clay stayed relaxed around the others who came to help, because nearly all were quiet, did not suck his energy, were content to share his space and be there for companionship and physical help. Only now can I put my finger on what was going on. In this realm I was sorely inadequate and unqualified. How do you get qualified to watch your child suffering and dying? I can only hope my physical help and presence and my love allowed him the time to complete his work. I know I sapped his strength, but I so wanted to hold on to him.

Thank God for his animals and plants. What a wonderful exchange of love and light. That must be what I am missing so now! The energy!

Our friends continued to take him to Tulsa for doctor's visits, for chemotherapy to try to keep the Kaposi's from overwhelming Clay, to pick up the strong medication Vancamyin for his newly diagnosed lung disease..Rhodococus Equii, to come for quiet visits. The doctor explained to me that Clay's lung infection was very rare and that they rarely survived 6 months with it…he beat that time frame by about 6 months..but it eventually took its toll on him.

I have pages and pages of notes with words jotted down so I wouldn't forget important things that happened…especially during the 6 months prior to Clay's death. It's like trying to describe a nightmare. It is not possible to convey the fear, panic and horror you felt while experiencing the nightmare. I remember that nightmare every day, and I remember glimpsing the nightmare in Clay's eyes. I am haunted by it. I guess that's why I have hesitated to go on with the story. I want to tell the story for Clay and for other individuals and families who have experienced the same battles..different actors, different locations..but the same results. I want the world to know about the nightmare of AIDS, I want them to be aware that their sisters, brothers, sons, daughters, co-workers, fellow churchgoers and neighbors may be experiencing that nightmare. They need compassion, understanding, prayers and help. My words to those experiencing the damned drama is to let you know that you will be strong enough; you do have enough love to endure; you and your dying one can wrestle this demon together. You are signed up for combat duty. You will not be prepared for the battles. They are not like you imagined. But, you can be "girded with hope and assurance" that the spirit of God is there in the midst of the sickness and suffering.

Your cries for help and relief do not go unheard. Physical healing does not happen. Our loved one, our Clay, had been undergoing a long healing process from within. When he died, his body was rotten, but his spirit and soul were clean as a newborn's....I could see it in his eyes. We felt it in his communications and philosophies. He became the teacher...the rabbi. He had 80-year old wisdom. Time was passing quickly.

I am going to have to tell about the days from the spring of 1993, through the long hot summer, and through autumn, Thanksgiving, and Christmas, until Clay left us on January 10, 1994. Forgive me if I sound maudlin or dramatic. It was maudlin and dramatic. The days and nights were wonderfully horrible. What? Wonderful because we were together and we still had Clay. Horrible because he was dying a horrible death while still so alive. Here goes.

The farmhouse we were living in was alive with activity, and swarmed with vermin. We were renting a "remodeled" old farmhouse with lots of holes from the outside walls into the house. The floor covering was deep shag pile of brownish-orange color...I think it was supposed to be burnt orange, but was filthy from the beginning...thus the brown color. We cleaned that carpet before our dogs and cats moved in, and were horrified at the black filth it picked up. We asked the landlord about it..had there been animals in there before? Had they cleaned it since then? "No" and "yes" were the answers. If you are familiar with animals, you will know that they will put their mark where other animals have been. So, guess what went on in our house!? Needless to say every time we cleaned the carpet, we pulled up more and more filth.

Why do I mention the holes and the carpet? Combine the smells of mouse droppings, dogs, wet carpets, and combine them with the smells associated with the terminally ill, and you will get the idea. Clay spent much of his time and energy washing bedclothes and his clothes, and trying to clean up after his animals. He loved them so..and he loved me. He was trying to keep me from having to deal with so much.

This bad scenario was more than offset by Clay's ability to make that house into a home. He arranged the furniture and hung his paintings. He filled the rooms with tasteful porcelain and copper bowls overflowing with sachets and silk flowers. He planted and grew plants and flowers inside and out. He shared his books and music, and his knowledge of those books and music, with us. He used his camera and took pictures of all the cattle, birds and squirrels sharing our little homestead with us.

While Clay was still mobile, he would drive his little red VW Rabbit into town and investigate. He joined the local college's workout facility and continued to swim on a regular basis. He roamed the countryside and enjoyed the simplicity of the woods surrounding the river and creeks. He continued to read, learn and observe. We had stimulating conversations and arguments. He had experienced and learned so much.

Clay's medical regimen, necessities and appointments combined with his excursions, my job and our housekeeping duties, made for some long days. We had a little difference in our sleep habits. He had not changed since he was a kid. And I had not changed since I was a kid. He was nocturnal. I am diurnal. He wandered around in a daze until about 11 a.m. and woke up about 11 p.m. I wandered around in a daze after about 10 p.m., but woke up about the time he had just settled in for a long snooze. His nightly wanderings and activities really affected my need for 8 hours of rest. Knowing that our time together was limited helped us to make concessions—sometimes very grudgingly. Understanding each other's idiosyncrasies, many of which we shared, created a good home life. We were alike in our love of music and learning. We shared an interest in the "world". Clay was very political...very liberal..very radical. No one had a chance to differ with Clay. He would override what a person thought he believed and knew by exerting the pure force of his personality. He studied every facet of the political, religious and social worlds and then would swarm everyone with the power of the knowledge he had gained. I listened and expanded my horizons, soaking up new ideas, and joining in the movements to help the sick and needy. My friends began calling me a classic "bleeding heart liberal". What else can you be when you are living with a gay son dying of AIDS in a world wishing the worst on both of them? Clay had to fight..and I tried to join right in.

The "mother lion" instinct to protect her cubs and fight their battles does not die easily. This primal protective instinct is ever lurking in a mother's heart and soul. When the cubs are hurt or in danger, all of those defending mechanisms are on full alert. It was the same with all four of my "cubs", but never stronger than during this battle against overwhelming odds. This cub had strayed outside of our territory and had returned mortally wounded. The pride gathered around him in an effort to shield him from further damage and to try to save his precious life. The mother lion in me urged me to sharpen my claws, build up my reserves, and to prepare to fight the battle with this prodigal cub. Our fortress was the old farmhouse in the hills of eastern Oklahoma, and our reserves were only determination and hope. When Clay was faced with mortal danger—a death sentence—the survival instinct which God has implanted in all living things roared to the forefront of our lives. Looking back, I see that we, mostly Clay, overcame events and emergencies with almost supernatural strength. Those who are fortunate enough not to have walked this type of nightmare path cannot appreciate the inner resources a being has when faced with the specter of a rotting body and difficult death.

I was awed and amazed to observe those who had a death sentence hanging over them living LIFE and grabbing new experiences with both hands. Clay never quit learning, dreaming, achieving. He never quit enjoying nature, listening to beautiful music, swooning over magnificent art. I could not quit or give up. Clay did not allow that. He encouraged and pushed me to live with him… to keep learning and loving. It was not easy to watch him desperately cramming all the life he could into his experience before the curtain came over those wonderful blue eyes. The heart that I have left cries, "If I only could have done more."

DAY TO DAY SURVIVAL

My first contacts with persons affected by HIV and AIDS were in 1987 and 1988. The share and support group in Ponca City was started by an older, loving couple whose only son had AIDS. When I found out that Clay had AIDS, I searched around and found the Green Country Mental Health Clinic of Ponca City, who recommended this support group. I remember how important it was to protect the identity of anyone who attended such a group. We were all open to all sort of problems at that time: loss of jobs and friends being the most obvious. Because the medical community had not really pinpointed how the virus was spread, anyone associated with the virus was subject to disassociation. You know, I heard once that they should put people with HIV/AIDS in colonies, like lepers once were. I probably heard this from my family. This first support group and the mental health clinic were the first sources of information for me about the disease. The Department of Human Services, state and federal, had printed some pretty informative booklets, with basic information. These booklets are still available and still informative, and should be mandatory curriculum in public schools and college campuses. During this learning time in Ponca City and in Tulsa, I became aware then that not only were they afflicted with a disease which limited their time on earth, but they were usually on a strict timetable for taking medications. In Long Beach I noticed a curious ritual: watch alarms sounding and pill boxes emerging for doses of mysterious medicines. Before, after and during mealtimes, pills would be dosed out on the table and taken religiously. Taking regular medication became not only a way of life, but a way TO life.

Clay and the army of those fighting this nasty little virus were voraciously gleaning information from medical journals, newspapers, libraries, and their own networking. Whenever they heard of some new diet, medication or treatment, they would hone in on it and share its results. Most were only a temporary respite, but offered hope. When the drug AZT became available (but not without a battle with the FDA), AIDS patients got their first real glimmer of a possibility of relief. It was very expensive and had side effects. Clay and others determined to live gained access to the drugs and information they needed and created a regimen for living. This regimen became a lifeline. I'm sure that only those whose lives are sustained by medications can understand this lifestyle.

I was increasingly uneasy about my ignorance in the area of what medications treated what infection or condition and how and when they were to be taken. The identity and importance of Clay's medications were evident, but he seemed to jealously guard that secret. I suspect he may have been trying to spare me in some way. On the other hand, I remember his remarking to me one day, "Mom, this is MY disease." And this was HIS walk. He had by trial and error, through suffering and pain, developed a plan which kept him alive and allowed him to have a fairly good quality of life. As Clay became weaker and frailer, I still could not get him to share the secret of the medications. Only when we were in the last two months did he allow me to make a list of drugs and which disorder they treated. The nightmare was coordinating those which must be taken with meals with those which should not be taken with food, and those which must be taken at bedtime and those which must be taken when the patient first awakens. Then there were to medications to combat the nausea and diarrhea caused by the drugs he took to stay alive. It was a race to stay ahead of the opportunistic diseases lurking and waiting to pounce on Clay's delicate system.

All the while Clay was working at staying alive, I was still working to help put food on the table and pay the rent. Clay had income through his Social Security disability and Medicaid, and that combined with my income paid our rent, groceries, car payments, dog care, and the medications which were not covered by Medicaid. I am unsure as to the exact figures and numbers which were involved in the Medicare and Social Security programs, but my memory is that there were limitations placed on how many and what type prescription they would cover. Recipients of these programs were allowed only three medications per month. Patients with HIV/AIDS take a multitude of prescription medicine in addition to all of the over-the-counter drugs, vitamins and other aids to assist them in staying alive. Medical benefits paid under the only programs available paid for hospital stays, up to a limited amount of days, doctor visits, chemotherapy up to a certain limit. Trying to set up a budget for financial survival would have been impossible and discouraging. In times like these you just keep moving, robbing Peter to pay Paul, and working hard. Clay knew how to budget and knew where each penny of his income must go. The struggle regarding finances took a lot of precious time and energy. It is a credit to Clay's ingenuity and survival instinct that our finances did not get out of hand. Maybe they did…I was just too numb to put too much importance to money or lack of money..whatever we were doing had to work.

We had no choice. I had one friend who will remain in my grateful heart forever who would supplement my income periodically when we just plain ran out of cash for groceries and gas. Thank you, friend, for all of those out-of-the blue contributions.

THE LAST DAYS

The spring and summer of 1993 were spent going back and forth to the cancer clinic in Tulsa for chemotherapy, as well as visits to the doctor and the journey to the druggists to get medication. Dr. Beal had us on a "mercy" regimen and was allowing us to charge some of Clay's drugs with a certain druggist, probably knowing full well that they might not get paid. Who says charity and caring are dead? Clay was using a cane and his legs and feet were swollen from the effects of the Kaposi's lesions. The lesions lessened in intensity from the chemotherapy and seemed to dry out. This cancer was under control externally but Clay and Dr. Beal knew internally the HIV had taken over and the Kaposi's were the least of Clay's worries. As we all know, chemotherapy may be killing cancer, but it further weakens the immune system..and Clay did not have much left. His T-cell count was nearly zero, but he kept going. He experienced a lot of nausea and weakness and loss of hair. In between these sessions, he was pretty much his old self. The staff at the cancer center were so supportive, and the room where the patients were receiving treatments were as pleasant as possible. The drives there and back allowed us some peaceful times to visit.

During late summer of 1993, Clay became noticeably weaker and was suffering considerable discomfort and difficulty in getting around. The pain medications allowed him to sleep more, but compromised his ability to maintain control of his medications. We needed help dispensing medications and meals while I was at work. I needed to be home with him but had to go to work. Dr. Beal and his staff went into what I call "the final days" mode and became tender and supportive. He prescribed Home Health Care and his office was always available for consultations. I was beginning to panic. I knew we were walking up on dying, and I wanted to get a handle on what I was supposed to do. I did not know how to help my son die. I had not been too hot on helping him live.

Clay and I were both shocked at his deteriorating condition. I practically screamed to Dr. Beal, "What happened all of a sudden?" He replied that the HIV had finally taken over and everything was failing. Clay stopped his chemotherapy. Getting in and out of the house and car and into the hospitals and clinics was excruciatingly painful for him. We had to simplify and try to make things as comfortable as possible. Emergencies became normal. Clay's system would become so debilitated that we would have to travel to Tulsa to St. John's hospital for transfusions. Each visit required going through the Emergency Room and checking in, which was a nightmare for someone as sick as Clay. He always handled the waits and delays like a gentleman. He empathized with the hospital workers and always started up a conversation with them to put them at ease. Bless his heart.

Have you experienced blood transfusions given to those who are trying to stay alive? It is so intense. Life blood. Clay's veins were closed up and knotted from all of the injections of medication and the transfusions took hours. We spent many nights isolated at the end of a hospital floor getting the life saving fluid. It seemed cold in those halls, but it was kind of a relief for Clay to be in capable, professional hands for a while. And we got some extra medications while there! This just added to our supply of medications. Clay felt so much better the next few days that it seemed worth it. When you are getting down to counting the days you have to live, you will endure almost any procedure which will prolong those days. It came to a point when Clay was too weak to make those trips, and Clay's clock began to wind down.

The first home health care team to help us came from the local hospital. Clay's pain level required large doses of morphine, literally more than the law allowed, and the workers were almost anal about dosing him. They were concerned that he was abusing the drug. The hospital sent out a morphine pump with their health care workers, which promptly malfunctioned in the middle of one evening. Clay called them and they advised him what to do. This did not work, and he endured a long painful night. The next day they brought out another pump, which malfunctioned in the middle of the night. This time he used his "spring creek" ingenuity and worked his way into the line and administered his own medication from the pump with a syringe. The hospital was horrified and chastised Clay for his actions, and took the pump away. We called Dr. Beal and he engaged another Home Health Care team and instructed them how to administer the pump, advised them of the seriousness of Clay's deteriorating condition, and how to care for him.

Clay and I got together with the Home Health Care ladies and made up a timetable for administering drugs, medications, and vitamins. Vitamins…now that was optimism. The will to survive…he still wanted a healthy diet and wanted to take his vitamins.

I still have a copy of the chart which was a timetable for administering medications. Clay sat down with me and explained the dosage and we reduced it to a chart:

Early AM (before 4 a.m.), before eating; Mid Morning; Noon; Afternoon; P.M.; Late P.M.; Bedtime (8 p.m.). His "Meds" Oramorph—30 mg.—three times a day; Videx—100 mg.—twice a day; Diflucan 100 mg—once a day; Sulfatrim—800 mg—once a day with LOT OF WATER; Zovirax—800 mg.—once a day; Biaxin—500 mg—twice a day; Lorazepam—2 mg.—one every 6 hours; Tamazepam—30 mg. At bedtime; Zoloft—as needed. My notes: "X" off when medications given. This little chart really helped. I could carry a copy with me in case we had to go to the emergency room, and I handed it to the nurses when we checked in. I think it helped them, too.

Clay helped educate the home health aides and nurses about his condition, how he should be handled, how to protect him and themselves. They were lucky that their first AIDS patient was so knowledgeable and willing to share his experience and knowledge with them. They enjoyed Clay's sense of humor and admired his intellect. He would share his love of books and music with them and told them a lot about his life. They not only ministered to Clay's needs, but worked around the dogs. Everyone worked around the dogs. Those dogs were Clay's lifeline. He needed the affection ,warmth and acceptance of Annabelle and Camille. They were just so connected. He spoiled them and they in turn smothered him with love. They slept with him until the last few days before he went to the hospital and was in such pain from the Kaposi's lesions.

The health care workers and the friends from the Green Country AIDS Coalition came in during the day and visited with Clay. Home Health Care came twice a day, once for medications and once for meals. I was so relieved that they were coming in. The friends from Green Country AIDS Coaliltion would take Clay to Tulsa for doctor's appointments or chemotherapy or to pick up medications. When he became too weak to walk without help, our helpers would just come visit and soothe him..and helped with meals. He loved them, and I appreciated them. When we took him to the hospital in the middle of the night before he died, some of them never saw him again. I think it must be very hard on workers like these wonderful, tender people. They develop a relationship with a person during the most intimate and intense part of their lives…their dying. These people were an integral part of Clay's last contact with life. And then…he's just gone. And they are left.

I cannot go further into this tale without mentioning my friends Louise and Bill, friends of the family who stood quietly in the background, Louise calling in her calming voice, and creating beautiful afghans for all of us. She and her unselfish husband made it their goal during our 30+ year friendship to acknowledge each child and grandchild by creating something special for them. Despite a full-time job, a husband, and raising her own two boys, Louise would weave beautiful afghans and give them to each of us. She would never take payment and would make sure she had an idea of the colors we wanted. She created Clay and me two beautiful afghans in 1993. Clay's had bright oranges and greens, a vibrant design, and was soft. He loved it. This afghan warded off the chills and gave him comfort when he was so miserable. They became our "security blankets" and we could snuggle under them, remember my friend's love, and feel shielded from the world we were in. The relationship with these friends began when Clay, Matt, and I moved to Oklahoma with my second husband. They were only 3 and 4 years old, and she was expecting her first child while I was expecting my first child with my new husband. So, this friendship has lasted through many changes in our lives. They were always there, always concerned. Later, you will see just how important this friendship became.

During the late summer of 1993, Clay's father came to visit for the first time in a few years. We had not been married since 1962, and he had remarried and had two beautiful daughters. He had been divorced a few years at this time. His one daughter was out on her own, and the other was beginning college. Clay had established contact with his father's family in Fort Worth, and his grandmother had been support-ive and had provided him with funds from some of the money he would have received as an inheritance. I think they sometimes thought we were pulling the wool over their eyes and just trying to get money from them. Clay's dad was very suspicious about giving us money. I overheard Clay in some pretty sad conversations with his father, liter-ally begging for money. I told him to quit begging. We could make it. He did not know how seriously ill Clay was until he visited that sum-mer day. Clay had maintained a very healthy and bright look during most of his illness, but by the time his dad came, he was visibly deteri-orating and walked, moved and had begun to look like an old man. When his father came in the door, he looked, stepped back out the door onto the porch in shock, and said , "Oh, my God, he looks like an old man". I think he finally realized Clay wasn't faking it, and was dying. I hope they had a good visit.. it was almost too late. Clay talked him into getting him an expensive bicycle. He never stopped longing for his father's support.

While Clay was working hard at living, what was happening to the rest of the family? His brother, Matt and Matt's daughter Del, had just returned to Texas after the military. Matt was in the process of establishing an optometry practice and trying to come back and forth to help. Del was an impressionable teenager—about 14—and looked very much like Clay. They shared the blonde hair, olive complexion, and big blue eyes. She was very close to Clay...just like her Daddy was. Matt and Clay were full brothers...13 months apart...and we had been through a lot together, even before I married Dan and Annie's father.

Dan, Clay's younger brother, and his wife Shelly, had moved to Houston, and were working and trying to come back and forth to help when they could. When Dan and Shelly made their wedding plans for July of 1993, they planned for Clay to be able to come, but he missed this beautiful event, too. And, once again, a momentous occasion in one of his sibling's lives was overshadowed by his illness. Shelly was actively supportive of all of us, and I know was a great comfort to Dan. She and Dan brought a lot of hilarity and fun into the household when they showed up. When the whole crew showed up, Clay just doubled over with laughter. They all entertained each other..and me. You have to admire the partners of the children who are in the midst of a long-playing crisis. They bear the brunt of a lot of intense situations. Shelly was exceptionally supportive (and exceptionally silly) and related well with Clay.

Annie, Clay's younger sister, was in Oklahoma City. She, too, had a demanding job, and was working at having a life. She and her boyfriend, Van, were both working and trying to come back and forth to help. In October, when Clay's condition began to worsen, Annie began coming over to Muskogee and Tahlequah on week-ends, most of the time with Van. I had a lot of admiration for this young man, who was very MALE, a veteran of Desert Storm, and just getting to know Annie. Talk about the baptism of fire. He was confronted with the dying brother of his new girlfriend, who not only had AIDS but was gay. And he still stuck around.

All of the kids were deeply affected by the turmoil. Their relationships, their jobs, their friendships, their time and their finances were stressed for several years. These were years in their lives which should have been devoted to developing their own lives. Their outlooks on life changed. New value structures were developed as we dealt with alienation from family members and some segments of society. I was constantly in a state of change trying to get into some sort of position to be able to deal with everything, and they were hovering on the fringes, moving me back and forth, and never, never did they express anger at me for the burdens I put on them. I am so very thankful for their sacrifices. And I am so very grateful that they all stuck together and supported Clay. What a team! I am so proud of them.

Thanksgiving of 1993 Dan and Shelly flew in from Houston to Oklahoma City. Annie picked them up at the airport and they visited, then she and Van brought them over to Muskogee and Tahlequah for turkey and dressing. Matt and Del drove up from Dallas, and the whole crew came to my apartment for turkey and dressing. Matt and Del stayed one night with Clay at the farmhouse, the other kids stayed at my apartment..and we cooked. It was bitterly cold and we had received some snow.

Clay was unsteady on his feet and Annie and Dan's father had made him a unique walking cane. He and the dogs arrived with Matt and Del on Thanksgiving Day at the apartment. He was using the cane and had on a maroon cardigan and a big, longcoat, and was in a festive mood. The apartment was not very big, and these were big boys, but we all enjoyed each other. We had come to grips that Clay's days were dwindling, and the kids decided to give him some of his Christmas gifts early. As I remember..they gave him lap blankets, long underwear, a couple of jaunty caps to wear over his bald head…my memory fails me on the details. It was poignant. We knew it was the last Thanksgiving we would have Clay. He knew it, too. Being together had become very important. It was awful. Clay tried to enjoy the meal, but the smells and taste of food just made him nauseous. He was so fatigued, but his humor was intact. They entertained each other into the night.

Matt and Dell took Clay back to Tahlequah in his little red VW Rabbit, and Shelly, Dan's wife, and Van, Annie's boyfriend, volunteered to follow them to be sure that little car made it. The temperature was down into the teens, dangerously cold. We expected them back at my apartment by 10:30 or so, and when they didn't show, we decided they had stopped somewhere to eat or something. By midnight, we became worried and Dan left to look for them. The stretch of highway between Muskogee and Tahlequah in the middle of the night on a holiday had few places to call for help.. and did not have much traffic. They all returned about 30 minutes later…Shelly and Van were chilled to the bone. A belt had broken on Van's car and they had been walking back toward Muskogee…which was about 15 miles from the point they broke down. They had walked about 5 miles before Dan found them. We were horrified but grateful they were not seriously hurt. The emergencies would not go away, and none of them fell away from the fight.

I have spoken about Clay's appearance. In the fall of 1992, when he came to eastern Oklahoma, he still had his stature, his hair, a fairly clear complexion, and had been spared the Kaposi's lesions on his face. They were beginning to become more numerous, but he looked fairly tanned and healthy. He was still swimming some and riding his bicycle, and looked anything but dying. He was very handsome and his manner belied his condition, even though he was in pain from his radiation treatments and other conditions. He did not begin to show the results of his long battle until about June 1993… 6 months before he died. The chemotherapy for the Kaposi's and the strong medication he took for his lung infection finally made him lose his hair. He immediately acquired a collection of "funky" hats and wore them or a bandana. He still worked in the yard with that bandana on. I would come home from work, and he would be sitting on the swing on the front porch, sweating from trying to work in the yard..I don't think he viewed it as work. He loved making things bloom and grow. So, he directed me on how to give them benevolent and effective care. I dug, he directed. The results were beautiful. His friends from the Green Country AIDS Coalition would come over and bathe and trim the dogs, mow the lawn and help around the house in addition to taking him back and forth for treatments and driving him around for tours of the country-side. He even rode the bicycle with a Groshong in his chest (a device implanted in his chest for administering medications) and KS lesions all over his legs. I was horrified, but he was not giving up on living. So, he maintained his appearance until about August, and then just fell apart. His mind remained active, his intellect and humor intact..until the end. He was so sensitive about his looks…but stayed beautiful to me.

Clay's comfort became an issue. The edema caused by the lesions and the lesions themselves kept Clay in pain all the time, and it was essential that he have a comfortable bed. Once again Clay took command and took a jaunt to a furniture store and picked out one of the most com-fortable (and expensive) mattress sets in the store. I was wringing my hands over the expense, but he knew he could not survive on the futon he had been sleeping on for years. With the addition of a foam egg crate cover, he was able to have a semi-comfortable place to stay. We thought about getting a hospital bed, because he was beginning to lose his equi-librium and had difficulty in pushing himself out of bed. We also began looking into getting a portable toilet, wheel chair, and walker..just anything which would help keep him mobile and out of the hospital ..and protect him from falling.

There are legal issues involved in dying. When a person becomes incapacitated and unable to handle his own physical and fiscal world, he must appoint or have available to him a "protector", if you will. The law provides protection for a person losing control of his life through Durable Powers of Attorney and Medical Directives. Clay had assisted many of his dying friends in preparing such documents while they were still in control. Knowing that you need to prepare and execute such instruments and actually going through the acts of relinquishing control of your life are two entirely different issues. When a person makes a will or signs a power of attorney or fills out a medical directive, they are admitting to themselves that they are not immortal. They have to face the hard fact that the last part of their lives will be dictated by someone else. Attending to the legalities was the worst part in Clay's final struggles.

When I had to go to the attorney, who was a friend, and draw up the papers appointing me guardian, I had to have Clay's permission, and it was so bad. I could not look Clay in the eye and felt that I was betraying him. He was looking to me to protect him and save him in some way, and when we had to fill out these papers, we had to admit we were beaten..the virus had won. Two weeks before Christmas, I knew I could no longer postpone the inevitable. I contacted Dr. Beal who sent me the following letter so that I could petition the courts to become Clay's guardian. I was particularly concerned that if we took Clay to the hospital, they would use "extraordinary measures" to keep him alive....and he had been through enough. His body was too damaged and frail to experience any invasive procedures. The saddest words written in a legal and impersonal way to protect I'm sure were dictated with much sadness. Clay had been one of the doctor's challenges..as if a medical team treating HIV needs challenges.

The letter:
December 13, 1993
To Whom It May Concern:

Clay Baker Shear has reached a point in living with AIDS where he suffers periods of confusion. This is in part related to his AIDS Dementia and in part related to medications. He is no longer competent to manage his own financial affairs.

Jeffrey A. Beal, M.D.
During the evening of December 14, 1993, I began working with Clay and talking with him about filling out the Advance Directive for Health Care, which contained a Living Will and directive for care when he became incapacitated. The directive appointed me or his brother or our friend Sara as a health care proxy and which was designed to state his wishes as to his treatment when he was no longer able to direct such care. Getting him to sign this directive was tantamount to wrestling an angel down. I had to be gentle but firm in insisting he go over the document with me, filling it out, and signing it..this was for his own protection. But, oh, this was such a final step. I wish we could have gone about this at an earlier time, but this was his call, and his life.

So there we were, two desperate souls, one wanting more than anything to stay alive and one wanting to save and hold her child, signing away his life. It was about three o'clock in the morning and I was piled up on his bed with him, holding the pen in his weak, wavering hand, as he wrote these words in the blanks, over and over…

"No embalming. Call Rabbi." "No code" *(My words added)*

Here's a sample of the eighteen statements he was adding these simple words to:

1. Living Will

a. If my attending physician and another physician determine that I am no longer able to make decision regarding my medical treatment, I direct my attending physician and other health care providers, pursuant to the Oklahoma rights of the Terminally Ill or Persistently Unconscious Act, to withhold or withdraw treatment from me under the circumstances I have indicated below by my signature. I understand that I will be given treatment that is necessary for my comfort or to alleviate my pain.

b. *If I have a terminal condition:*

(1) I direct that life-sustaining treatment shall be withheld or withdrawn if such treatment would only prolong my process of dying, and if my attending physician and another physician determine that I have an incurable and irreversible condition that even with the administration of life sustaining treatment will cause my death within six (6) months.

(2) I understand that the subject of the artificial administration of nutrition and hydration (food and water) that will only prolong the process of dying from an incurable and irreversible condition is of particular importance. I understand that if I do not sign this paragraph, artificially administrated nutrition and hydration will be administered to me. I further understand that if I sign this paragraph, I am authorizing the withholding or withdrawal of artificially administered nutrition (food and hydration (water).

This document was witnessed by our two good friends, Jane and Gloria.

On December 16th, 1993, I petitioned the Court to appoint me as Clay's guardian and announce to the world …

"That Clay Baker Shear is impaired by reason of his dementia, and that this impairment results in his inability to receive and evaluate information effectively, meet the essential requirements for his physical health and safety, and in his inability to manage his financial resources."

For Clay's protection, I had to notify him that I was doing this. This court action was completed on December 30th, 1993, 12 days before Clay died.

Why am I including these facts in this book? Because in the midst of the hell of walking through the valley of death, measures must be taken to protect the weak, sick and dying from the "system", good or bad. Our certain inalienable rights can sometimes cause us much suffering if we do not have an advocate. People in the medical field and institutions are set up to keep people alive, no matter what, unless there are guardians in place to allow the person to live and die with a modicum of dignity. And I was determined that Clay would be in control of those last moments, and that his wish to go with dignity would not be denied. These are not easy steps to take, and can be ignored because the person is going to die anyway..so what's the point? To me, an individual's right to die peacefully and in a manner that dignifies his life, is sacred. It was my sacred duty as Clay's mother and friend to make his transition from this earth as gracious as possible. The last steps of his walk were faltering, but we were determined that this last journey would be as full and forceful as Clay's life had been.

As far as the Directive is concerned, I literally had to hold it up and block a nurse from Clay's room to keep her from administering a treatment to Clay. We had expressed to the staff to just keep him comfortable and allow him to rest and communicate peacefully with his family, his friends, and his God. I kept the Guardianship Papers and Medical Directive in my purse at all times.

THE JOURNEY HOME

The two weeks before Christmas in 1993 were the longest, yet shortest of my life. The longest because we were literally wrestling with Clay to keep him comfortable, to get him back and forth from his bed to a comfortable place to sit, then finally just to get him comfortable. The shortest because it would soon be over, and we would not have Clay.

Clay was 6 ft. 4", and I am 5 ft. 3" and not endowed with a lot of strength, but we were determined that we could make it and that he could stay at home during his last days. The path from Clay's bed to the toilet was a short one, but became a dangerous and challenging trip. At first he could stumble along holding to the walls or using his cane and get to the toilet, but would often fall forward, and then we would struggle to get back to his bed. Sometimes when he was too weak, or I couldn't support him, he would crawl. In order to get back up on the bed I would have to get behind him as he grasped the sides of the mattress with both hands and arms. Then I would push with all my might and he would pull with his waning strength and we would wrestle him back up on that very high mattress. We knew we could not continue without help. This ritual was much flawed and I know it was hurting Clay. And did not help his dignity. I sent out the distress signal to the kids and told them what was going on. I finally admitted that it was excusable to miss work..or to put it more eloquently: "To hell with work." At this point nothing was more important that being with Clay and helping him through his last days. What I did outside of Clay's sphere no longer mattered. I had to be there. I felt terribly responsible. I don't know if I needed to be with Clay more than he needed me. Clay was working through this sad and final time on his own, but he needed our help. So, here came the kids. Annie took leave from her job..I guess her work didn't matter either at this point. And, she was the "point man" in Oklahoma City.   Clay had converted to Judaism and wanted an orthodox Jewish burial. Annie contacted Clay's synagogue in Oklahoma City and began getting the process for a Jewish burial. We had to make arrangements for a burial spot at a Hebrew cemetery, and because we were not Jewish, we needed to know just what it entailed.

Clay had given me his prayer book, his prayer shawls, his confirmation papers and some information and names, so that we could bury him in the manner he believed. Orthodox Jews do not believe in embalming, and it was our understanding they the body is to be buried within 48 hours. We were gathering this information while dealing with Clay's suffering and trying to stay alive. God bless Annie for her work. I know it wasn't easy.   Making this type of arrangement and the legal work made me feel like we were betraying Clay by admitting that he was going to die. But it had to be done.

The best part of the worst part was being there with Clay, having his presence. Watching him slip into the hands of death was like a bad dream. One night I slipped into his room and watched him in his sleep and the reality that he was dying finally gripped by heart. His mouth was open and his eyes fixed and he was breathing deeply with a soft gurgling sound. I slipped into my little cubbyhole and began writing his eulogy. It never was read at the funeral because they could not find it, but this scrawled letter written in the middle of the night and splotched with desperate tears tried to express my love for this boy.

"I Learned to Love from My Children

Not until I held my first child in my arms did I realize the depth of emotions which were embedded within the human spirit. Each child and each unique experience with each one brought forth the awareness

of the real meaning of love. All four children brought four completely different ranges of love and caring into our world.

But this is about Clay—our second child. I say "our"—I mean the whole family. Because Clay has changed all our lives and has made us all aware of the good and the bad in each one of us, and because of his experiences has made us broaden our sense of caring and fairness to our fellow man.

To put it in a few words, because of Clay's curiosity and his view of life, each person in his path of lime came to look at the world in a new and different light, whether we wanted to or not.

As a baby he was sweet and alert, undemanding and relaxed. As he grew, his curiosity about bugs and butterflies, and flowers and trees, and dogs and cats..made our walks *very* long. He wanted to know "why?" and "how?" and when he could read, he satisfied a lot of curiosity by reading. Clay and all the children were ornery and busy, health and rambunctious. They all have always had a "zest for life".

Clay's quest for this "zest of life" led him through some difficult times. His analytical mind, combined with his tenderness for life, love of beautiful things, and sense of justice put him on a path which led him into different worlds—into varied experiences. He embraced Judaism, after studying and experiencing other religions, because of Judaism's all encompassing philosophy of God and its call for caring, compassion and responsibility for others.

He was true to his own personal philosophies and stood his ground to be true to his own uniqueness.

This wonderful mind, his love of music and art, his sharing of himself with wounded and dying friends, his unholy sense of humor, his great, undying affection for his animals, his regard for the poor and suffering, his demand for political justice, his love of nature..made him a complicated, and often difficult, person, because there was never room for compromise.

We will never know what a wonderful experience he had in California and in his travels. We will never know about his loves and tribulations during the years he was away and searching, but he brought back to us some of the joy of them—and some of the depth of the experiences he had.

The one most important was his experience with the epidemic known as AIDS. He has brought it into our midst through his own personal walk with the disease, and caused us to stand up and look within ourselves and to examine our prejudices and beliefs. He has educated us in caring for others, by allowing us to care for him. He has bravely fought the battle for fairness and for good medical care for himself and others. He has "beaten the odds" in this disease several times, and suffered all the indignities imposed upon those who suffer from debilitating diseases..and emerged with dignity.

The essence of his being is being celebrated today and the passing of this soul will be celebrated by those meeting him who have gone before him…his grandmothers, grandfathers and friends..The loss of this light will be sorely missed by those still here..but the warmth of the fire he lit within each of us to pull from our own depth of resources, to serve, to love, to accept without judgement and prejudice—the coals he put beneath our feet and in our hearts, will continue to spread and change us and those we touch forever.

God bless you, my dear—

God blessed us all by letting us have you for a while."

In the days, months and years before this point, I had been confident that we were enough in control that we could keep Clay at home and keep him comfortable until he died. He wanted to die at home and told me several times he did not want to go back to the hospital. But, you know as Robert Burns expressed, "The best laid plans of mice and men, G'ang aft agly". We did not really have a plan, only a hope that we were strong enough and capable to carry such a burden to fruition. When pain takes over and the confusion and turmoil mix with the sounds and smells, and every well meant but unskilled touch causes more pain, then it is time to get to a place where skilled hands can give a little comfort.

The days before Christmas in 1993 were a jumble of deep sadness and a sense of emergency. All of the children and their partners came to the house prepared for the battle to keep Clay as happy and comfortable as possible and to spend his last moments with him. Reluctant to let him go! You bet! But watching him endure the indignities thrust upon him as he became less and less in control prompted us to pray for his relief. No. But, oh, we did not want to lose him. You do not know what to pray. Just give us strength, love, and wisdom, Lord. We are new at this, Lord. Guide our hands. Clay was new to this experience, too, but had been taking careful measures to clear the path for his journey Home.

He was a kind and thoughtful patient and kept his sense of humor while we tried to make him comfortable. We had to keep ourselves out of his way so that he could rest and sleep, but we had to remain alert for sounds of his trying to get out of bed when he needed to use the bathroom. He still wanted to be independent. Annie and Van came first and sent me packing to my apartment for a night and told me that they would hear a thump and Clay would have fallen trying to get to the potty chair, as he named it. When Van carried Clay to the bathroom, Clay looked up into his eyes and gleefully said, "Van, will you marry me?" The next day Matt, Del, Dan and Shelly came in to help. Christmas Day dawned.

I had checked in with Dr. Beal's office during the week before Christmas, and they had advised that Dr. Beal was taking a much-needed vacation the week after Christmas, but assured me that someone would be on call if we needed help. A doctor treating people with AIDS does not have a long, willing list of physicians to call upon, but we had no choice but to hope we would not need to call them. I also had to find out what we legally were required to do if someone dies at home.

Call an ambulance, have a doctor pronounce them dead. I could not even think that far ahead, but I had the information. This was too much reality and believe it or not, I was in denial. I did not think this moment would ever come. I wanted Clay to be without pain and to be rid of this awful experience, but this meant losing him to that everlasting sleep.

The kids were in a frenzy of service, dodging dogs, washing bed-clothes and dishes. They were trying to have Christmas and trying to stay sane. They were hovering near Clay to be there to speak with him, to hear him, to love him. One evening, Van, Annie's boyfriend, dropped quietly at my feet and whispered, "Ann, I don't mean to say anything hurtful, but I got some of Clay's pee on my foot while ago and won-dered..you know..if it is dangerous or anything." Bless his heart. This was so hard on him. I just told him that if anyone peed on his foot, he should probably wash it off, but that urine was not an agent to worry about. We had lots of boxes of gloves to wear, and the sounds of gloves going on and being pulled off were added to the cacophony of sounds in that busy household. We had bottles of alcohol and Lysol handy to clean up any accidental blood or stool spills. We had bleach by the kitchen and bathroom sinks, and washed dishes with a mixture of bleach and detergent.

Leslie, Clay's friend from high school and his "partner in crime" as he was growing up, had been coming over to visit with Clay. She and Clay were still mischievous and laughed for hours about their escapades. She brought him flower arrangements, visited with him, and then went out and cried. She was there for him and remained there and available to Clay and to the family until the end. Thanks Leslie, wherever you are. We began the search for Harold, although he had been gone for over a year. Clay was really disappointed in Harold's running away, but under-stood that some people just cannot handle the strain. He did not believe he would ever see Harold again.

Clay had an implant in his vena cava with three ports so that medi-cine could be infused into his body without injections. He no longer had viable veins for intravenous injections and had been sporting this device for some months. As his body deteriorated and his system lost its fluids, this implant became less stable. As we tried to help Clay around, we were very aware that we could knock this lose and feared what Clay would have to endure to re-attach the device should we do so. He did not need to undergo any invasive and painful procedures. Poor Clay. We were such neophytes! I know we made him uneasy watching us fumble around, and he gave us direction—sometimes he had to be very harsh and became impatient when we did not understand what he needed. He knew the drill. The health care workers came in for the last time Christmas day to give us a hand and to give us some professional help. We tried to share a little Christmas with them, and we did manage to have a Christmas of sorts. Clay had been observing Hanukkah, too, so we had the family nativity scene and the Star of David and the menorah displayed on the same table. We had shared gifts and cooked Christmas dinner. Truthfully, most of us do not remember the details of each day. We have blocked out many details. I have had to really sit down with each of the kids to ask them what they remember. It is very painful, but I hope it will help the healing. We do remember Matt sharing with Clay some of the brandy which was an ingredient of a "homemade" fruit cake. Even though Clay was not always completely alert, he took a swig, choked and coughed, and said gruffly and with his characteristically wicked smile, "Smooooth!"

Matt had set up his optometry office in Texas on the first of December, and one of his Christmas presents for Clay was a pair of violet-colored contacts. Matt told Clay it made him look like Elizabeth Taylor, and Clay felt "beautiful". Again, Clay's brothers and sister were living around his condition. They were taking care of themselves, their jobs, their homes and children, running back and forth, and watching their brother die a terrible death.

The kids remember many of the details of the last days, but admit they have blocked out a lot. I remember gratefully going to my apartment, bathing, making calls, and just resting. Then, I remember the call from Matt on the day after Christmas. "Mom, we dropped Clay and we are hurting him. We need to take him to the hospital." Boom. Five of them could not handle him. They were sore and aching from working with him. They knew I could do no more if they left to go back to their jobs. They had not given up, but they knew the reality.

For several days, the kids had been taking shifts of staying near Clay's bedroom to listen for him. One bedroom near him had a waterbed in it, but was really hard to climb out of in a hurry. So, Matt had taken the cushions off the couch, laid them on the floor next to Clay's bedroom door, and made a spot to spring from. During the last nights Clay slept on the couch, so that he could get up and down easier, and he did not have so far to fall. He was slipping in and out of reality, and although he sounded lucid at times and we had many conversations with him, he was losing control of his thoughts and actions. Basic individual drives and instincts try to override the physical condition. One of Clay's fears was always that he would have to wear a diaper and we would have to clean him up. Either by will or by grace he was not subjected to this type of indignity until the end. By the time he was losing control of his faculties, his system was dehydrated to the point that his trips to the bathroom were very limited. Clay still felt pressure in his bowel and felt the need to urinate and would try to get out of bed to get to the bathroom. He was too weak to even try to negotiate the portable toilet, but would try. He did not want to disturb anyone and was really too weak to call out. I bought him a little bell to ring, but he did not even have strength to ring it.

Therefore, the first notification we had that he was trying to get to the toilet was a loud thump as he hit the floor. We came to dread the sound, but developed the ability to get to Clay in seconds. It reminded me of early parenthood when you could bound out of bed and be ready for action at the slightest sound from baby's room. Clay and I had about

3 months of this drill, and then shared the experience with the kids. They were worn out.

It wasn't all a nightmare during those last days. The kids lovingly teased Clay as they were ministering to him. He was embarrassed when Annie would help bathe him, but she kidded him out of it. They were gentle and pleasant, and then I would catch them sitting in the other room gripping the arm of the chair staring into space. Instinctively, my children were caring for their wounded brother the way they would want to be treated if they were in his shoes. They traded time and energy with one another. They did things I could not do physically, and they allowed Clay to stay among the living. They teased him and shared with him and held him.

The day after Christmas 1993 was a Sunday. The health care workers, the doctor's office and the family had decided we could wait no longer, so we headed for the hospital in Tulsa, 60 miles away. Annie and Van took their car so they could go back to Oklahoma City. Dan and Shelly stayed at the house and began moving furniture. Matt went back and they worked cleaning and moving. Matt made a run to Texas to pick up the trailer and brought it back and they picked up furniture, moved some to my apartment in Muskogee, some in storage and took the rest to their homes or to be stored at the lake. We felt like vultures and were heavy with fatigue and sad hearts. Dan and Shelly took Annabelle and Camille to Houston with them to separate them from the trauma of losing Clay.

We had called ahead to Dr. Beal's office knowing he was out of town. The only doctor he could get to cover for him was a psychologist, but at least he could get us into the Emergency Room and into a room. We left Tahlequah late in the morning and arrived at the Emergency Room in the early afternoon, thinking we would go straight to his room and he could begin getting some professional care. But, as all people know who have to deal with hospitals, nothing was ready and the emergency room was full to capacity. Tulsa was in the middle of a flu epidemic and it was a holiday week-end. Clay was weak and sick and could hardly bear the strain of waiting. And I could not look Clay in the eye..and I could not let him out of my sight. I had promised him he could stay home. He had told me he did not want to go back into the hospital. I just wanted him to be comfortable and to be able to rest. We went through nearly the same process Clay and I had been through every time we checked in. This time it was different. He was coming in to die.

A bed in a cubicle had just been vacated and when the receptionist finally realized how ill Clay was an orderly arrived to escort us back there. It seemed so cluttered and public. Someone had thrown up on the floor. I was just desperate for Clay to begin receiving some professional care. The psychologist came back and visited with us and in about two hours we were moved to a room on the general hospital floor. I remember when we arrived. They were overloaded and not staffed to give round-the-clock care to someone who was bedridden. I had thought I could get a break and that there would be plenty of care. The frazzled but courteous nurse advised me that they were understaffed and someone needed to be there with Clay all the time. I was shocked and scared. Everyone had left town.

You know how God works through people, don't you? When I sat in the waiting room dealing with this problem, I gave a call to Dr. Beal's office and they gave me the number of Interfaith Ministries. I made one call for help. The next day people began showing up from Shanti, Interfaith Ministries, the Metropolitan ministries, churches, synagogues, and just general people who cared. They were gay and straight. They organized themselves into a schedule and began coming in 4 and 6 hour shifts day and night. Complete strangers...angels of mercy and love. I have one of their schedules: here are some of the names: Herb, Tim, Jim, Bill, Jason, Jay, Don, Randy, John Paul, Evelyn, Diane, Ken. Some of them walked from their homes or rode the bus in the middle of the night. They worked with my friends Bill and Louise, and later coordinated with Clay's friends Leslie and Harold. They were gentle and concerned and communicated with Clay by touch and speaking.

I brought Clay's favorite afghan and throws and pictures of his animals and favorite scenes and brought a little tape player for music. It did not run smoothly and was not beautiful and wonderful, but I cannot deny that Clay was surrounded by an aura of love. The room was alive with a positive charge of energy as Clay embraced his last walk in our physical world. Not only did Clay have escorts for this walk in his hospital room, but his escorts from his destination became active. Clay began the process of cleaning his soul and spirit for his trip home.

After about five days, Clay sat up and told me very firmly that he wanted to see his brothers and sister. His orders were: "I want to see Annie and Van, Danny and Shelly, Matt and Del". He needed them all here. He began to advise me to make sure all of our passports were in order for the trip. I had to retrieve his passport and documentation for travel from his belongings and give them to him, along with his prayer book, prayer shawl and yarmulke. Each day until all of the kids came back, Clay would anxiously ask me if all the passports were in order. One night we were visiting, and he was telling me about his visits from his grandmothers and grandfather Shear who were dead, I asked him where we were all going. He explained patiently and tenderly that I should not be alarmed. His passport was only one way, but ours was round trip. I asked him where we were going. And he looked surprised that I didn't know. His reply, "Jerusalem, of course". Of course. He was going Home with his God and all of His saints. When all of his brothers and sisters were gathered and he was assured that all of our papers were in order, he was satisfied that we were all prepared and safe for his trip.

Clay had a real tie with Matt's daughter Del. Clay and Del looked like father and daughter. They shared an olive complexion, blonde hair, blue eyes, and long lean build. He would rally when she came into the room and he would gaze at her. The last time Del came in, Del was dressed in blue which accented her eyes. Clay remarked, "You look flirty today!" He was concerned for Del as she grew up into this world full of temptations and pitfalls. I'm sure he was remembering his own turbulent adolescent days and the outcome of his deceit and excesses as he pulled her close to him with both hands and earnestly told her, "Be honest". He was warning a person he loved, so she wouldn't have to experience this hell.

During the last days and nights before Clay died, Clay's friend Sara, Bill, Louise and the other angels were witnesses to Clay's interaction with those who were going to escort him home. Sara had told me that once she had a dream about Clay. She asked me if we had a lot of relatives who had passed away. I told her that he had some great-grandparents and grandparents he loved who had died. She said she saw a lot of bright lights at the end of a path which Clay was on. I told her they must be all of the people he had helped live and then to die in California and Oklahoma. He was not going to walk that path alone.

One night Harold and I were keeping the vigil. This was not a quiet vigil. Clay was busy. I was on the right side of the bed and Harold was on the left side. Clay had been handing me the "bad stuff" and indicating that I should throw it away. He kept this activity going until he was ready. There was nothing bad left. He was healed. Healed from the inside. His body had given way, but his soul was clean and ready for the journey. And as a loving, caring son he took his precious energy to try to make sure his Mom was taken care of. I was on one side of the bed and Harold was on the other side. Clay kept taking my hands and trying to lift my arms over him. He did this several time and then exasperated with our confusion, repeated over and over, "Here, Harold....here." He was handing me over to Harold's care. I asked him if he wanted Harold to take care of me and he nodded. So, I let him stretch my arms over and past him to Harold's side. He was relieved knowing that responsibility had been passed on. We assured him that I was going to be okay, and that Harold would take over. We were all on a new journey and he and the angels were the tour guides.

Elisabeth Kubler-Ross's book *Death, the Final Stage of Growth,* which has chapters written by Rabbi Zachary I. Heller titled "The Jewish View of Death: Guidelines for Mourning", which helped explain how Clay had been developing his approach to his dying. Clay gave me this book to read so that I would know what he believed and his and Judaism's approach to this part of life. Some of Kubler-Ross's comments and summary preceding the first of these chapters helped me interpret and understand Clay's activities and beliefs during the last years. I will share some of them with you with Ms. Kubler-Ross's permission.

"*In the selection that follows, the author explains the rituals of the Jewish culture, set down in Jewish law, which provide for death with dignity and meaning—allowing the dying person to set his house in order, bless his family, pass on any messages to them he feels important, and make his peace with God. The meaningfulness with which these dictates of Jewish law are carried out, as in any situation, depends on the persons participating in the rituals as well as the degree to which the dying person's Jewish identify is integrated into his total life. But the prescribed procedures accompanying the dying of an individual of the Jewish faith and culture, if followed with meaning, give an outlet to the needs of the dying person.*"

Rabbi Heller states: "*Human mortality may not be denied, for death is the common end to all life. To the individual of traditional faith, death is not an end but a transition from one state of human existence to another. Yet, while we may be willing to accept the ultimate effect of this transition with equanimity, the process of dying is fraught with many anxieties that cannot easily be resolved.*"

One of my family members expressed to me that she did not see why Clay did not just kill himself, knowing what was ahead. Meaning..wouldn't it just be easier on him and the family? I know that most people who have HIV and other terminal illnesses have considered the option of suicide, and some act upon it. I know, too, that Clay had access to the formula for the combination of drugs and medications that could bring his suffering to an end. He had that combination in his possession. But Clay had converted to Judaism. He had converted in every way and not lightly. He had studied, prayed and counseled with the elders in the synagogue. He believed in the spirit and in the letter of the Judaic law. He believed in the sanctity of life within the framework of the Hallacha (the Jewish legal system).

Rabbi Heller refers to the following confessional as a "means of reconciliation with God":

"I acknowledge before you Lord My God and God of my fathers that both my healing and my death are in your hands. May it be Your will to heal me in a complete recovery. If, though, I do die, may my death atone for all my sins and transgressions that I have committed before you. Grant me a share in the world to come...."

When I read these words, I know why Clay's last years were so full of life. These were rules and laws he could understand and he had great respect for them. Clay let me know that his last days and his burial must be according to orthodox Jewish laws. We had the job of discovering just what we were to do to carry out his wishes in accordance with his beliefs.

Clay had given me the name of one rabbi who had helped him in his conversion to Judaism in Oklahoma City and some of his fellow believers in Norman at the Hillel Foundation. He had taken me to the synagogue in Oklahoma City and given me a tour of the Hillel Foundation in Norman. He had given some classes to students at the Hillel, as well as working as a janitor. Clay's little sister, Annie, who lived in Oklahoma City, took on the task of contacting that synagogue for help in arranging an orthodox Jewish burial. As many older siblings do, the boys had always considered Annie to be somewhat spoiled and irresponsible. Her actions and work in arranging for Clay's funeral while holding down a responsible job and taking care of her boyfriend's children, plus ministering to him and to me, should forever change that view.

We knew there was a time frame in which the body had to be buried and that the body was not to be embalmed. Clay told us he had to be buried in a Jewish cemetery. And Annie got to work. She contacted the synagogue and made arrangements to meet with the people who were in charge of the cemetery and the necessary ceremonies. She found out that they had a group of people who would prepare the body for burial and sit with the body before the burial. Annie called one of her friends who worked for a funeral home in Oklahoma City to get help in arranging for the body to be moved from Tulsa to Oklahoma City. She admonished them that he was not to be embalmed. The rabbi in Tulsa who visited and prayed with Clay during the last days gave us counsel and advice. The rabbi from Oklahoma City visited with Clay and gave him assurance. Annie located the cemetery and picked out a space under a tree in the cemetery in Oklahoma City. She learned that they had a special section for single people. She had to coordinate all of this while Clay was still living, so that when the end came, we could follow the Jewish laws and Clay's wishes. It was all in place, but it did not work out that way. The stigma of AIDS still was a part of this final ritual.

THE END

On about the eighth day of the hospital stay, I noticed a note to me posted on the bulletin board which was on the wall of the entrance to Clay's room. This note was from the hospital patient discharge worker saying he must see me. When we talked he wanted to know if I had plans for Clay's care after he left the hospital and did I know where he would be taken. I was astounded and replied in my cynical, smart aleck way, "To Heaven, I imagine". He was not really satisfied with this answer and patiently explained that Medicare only covered ten days in the hospital and that time was nearly up. I proceeded to fall apart and called the doctor to help. I expressed very loudly and strongly that I did not want him moved and hurt. What was the point? They asked me if I could afford the hospital charges if he was not covered. I didn't bat an eye and said, "Of course, I can afford it. Don't worry about it. Just keep him here and keep him comfortable". But I called Dr. Beal in a panic.

I was assured that Clay would be kept comfortable and I did not have to worry about moving him. They did offer the extended care floor which he could be moved into if he continued to live. I again begged and pleaded that he not be moved. I just wanted him tucked in and allowed to be peaceful and complete his preparations.

That brings to mind another memory. As Clay was ridding himself of the baggage of his life, he was also shedding any type of clothing which might touch his body. So, here was this young man as bald and as naked as a new born baby. In fact he looked like the baby I first held in my arms 33 years before. His starkly blue eyes looked so innocent and sweet, and as they looked into mine, I felt as if they were imploring me to save him. The strings to my heart were breaking as his heart kept up the valiant struggle for survival. Clay's mind and heart were still alert as his body died. Those are the worst moments. Never to see that flicker of light and intelligence in his face, never to feel the warmth of his hands, or the sounds of his laughter. And he did not want to leave.

Clay was still definitely gay. Dr. Beal and came in a few days before Clay died dressed in a pink shirt and tie, looking quite handsome. Clay pushed himself up and just grinned and said "Hi". He still appreciated a handsome man. When you have been hovered over by just relatives and caretakers, it must be a relief to see youth and vibrancy bounce into the room. After this visit I stopped Dr. Beal to ask what we were looking at. He said with tears in his eyes: "I thought if anyone could beat this, Clay could". What a hard thing for these doctors, watching hundreds of young people disintegrate before their eyes. I salute their fortitude and willingness to deal compassionately and effectively with this unknown virus and its inexplicable course with each person.

I cannot complete this narrative without giving thanks to God for His grace, strength and protection. I felt the presence of God's spirit throughout the whole ordeal with Clay. And on those dark days when we were in the depths of despair, Clay and I both sang the Psalms and recalled the comfort of the scriptures. Those last days in the hospital I spent many hours walking and singing those simple little Bible School songs I had learned over 50 years ago at the Methodist church we had grown up in. The grand uplifting hymns, "Balm in Gilead", "A Mighty Fortress", "O God Our Help in Ages Past", "Abide With Me", and the simple words of "Jesus loves me, this I know" which I sang to Clay during the last gray hours.

Beginning on Sunday morning before Clay died on Monday night, Harold and I were afraid to leave his side. We spoke to him and sang to him, and I prayed with him. In the deep dark dawn before he went into a coma-like state, I said, "The Lord is my Shepherd.." and Clay rallied and said, "I shall not want." We were truly in the Valley of the Shadow of Death. We were, like all "spectators" sitting with our loved ones as they struggle on that plain between life and death, concerned that he was comfortable but anxious that he be relieved of all that pain. It's that horrible span of time of unspoken anxiety. Knowing that death was imminent we were in a way hoping for it to be finished, but dreading the loss. It occurred to me that Clay probably felt the same way. I laid across the bed whispering to Clay that it was okay to go ahead and finish the trip. He was not ready, and looked up at me and begged, "Mom, I don't want to die". Dear God.

Monday morning, after a long, busy night , I stepped out to make a few calls and to get a cup of coffee. I called Bill and Louise and Tim, one of the wonderful gay young men we had met, agreed to come in the late afternoon, and Clay's soul mate, Sara was scheduled to come in early afternoon. I knew he would be in good hands.

When I came back to Clay's room, they had turned Clay and hurt him so badly that he withdrew into the comfort of a deep sleep..his last here on this old earth. I was reluctant to leave because I wanted to be there when he left. The hospital offered some sleeping rooms to Harold and to me. I let Harold go and at the urging of Clay's helpers and angels decided to take the trip back to Muskogee to clean up and sleep. Sara came in, lit candles and played soft and beautiful music , prayed and communed quietly with Clay as his spirit began to drift away.

As soon as Sara left and I was out of the picture, hospital personnel swept in and moved Clay to another floor, to a new room on another floor, completely against my wishes and without consulting any of the family. I know it hurt him even more and I hope he was beyond the pain. I hate to think that his last hours were so difficult. Louise and Bill were there when this went on, and took charge. Soon after, I understand that Clay just took his last breath and died. Louise made the call to me at my apartment about 7:00 to tell me that he was gone.

I thought I would be ready, but I could not even find my clothes, my purse, my keys, my coat. I had to call the kids. I had to drive back to the hospital to be with the body so that the funeral homes could transfer him to Oklahoma City for preparation for burial. The phone rang and my niece called to say that she and my sister were coming to the funeral. I had to tell them not to come and that Clay did not want them there. I did not want them there. They had not been there when he was alive, so what was the point? I was hysterical by this time and called Matt to call my sister's family to tell them to stay away.

I finally accumulated what I thought I needed and drove numbly, and very fast, to the hospital. It was a clear, cold night. We had been so fortunate that we never had ice or snow during these trips to the hospital and doctors' offices in Tulsa. I remember turning into the hospital parking lot and seeing my friends Bill and Louise waiting for me next to their van. That's when they told me he had been moved to another room and another floor. I couldn't believe it! I was surprised to find Clay's half sister and her boyfriend who had flown in from Las Vegas standing in the hall. They had missed being with Clay when he was still alive and were devastated. We couldn't find Harold. He had taken a walk. Leslie came.

My friends took me to the room and left me to get my last hug and kiss. It seemed unreal that my little boy, my grown son was just...no longer. I would never talk with him again. It was quiet and antiseptic..all I could say was, "I'm so sorry, Clay. I'm so sorry I couldn't save you. I'm so sorry." I have never felt so helpless.

It was about 10:30 or 11:00 in the evening and the hospital personnel and funeral home attendants were anxious to get the body out of there and to get on with the transport. We had made all arrangements with them and they had coordinated with the team of people at the synagogue. Yet, the Tulsa team for the funeral home explained that Clay had to be embalmed, that it was State law that someone with AIDS had to be embalmed.

I was in such a state that I could not argue, but was definitely confused. That reasoning is exactly opposite to what I already knew about invasive procedures for a person who had a communicable disease. I certainly did not think the synagogue would approve it unless tradition was overridden by the law. I was wrong. The committee had decided they did not want to touch the body unless it was embalmed. They did not call Annie. They did not communicate with me. They did not communicate.

I remember watching them wheel Clay away and felt assured that when he got to Oklahoma City, the committee at the synagogue would clean and bind the body according to custom as they had explained to me . I thought they would sit with the body the morning of the service on Wednesday at the funeral home. Again . . no matter what the plan, no matter what the circumstances and how stressful the situation may be, people just do not do what they promise. Clay's last wishes: to die at home and not to be embalmed were overridden by circumstances and ignorance and the fear of AIDS.

For anyone who goes through this ritual of burying their loved ones, you will understand this next statement. I have visited with each of my children at length trying to get the chronology of events before and after Clay became so very sick. It seems that we have all blocked out many of the details. We are remembering the high points and the good moments, but can't remember just how everyone got where they were at certain critical points. We just draw a blank. It was too hard on everyone and it is too intense to try to pull from the protective covering of our subconscious. We have spun a cocoon around that time and some things will just remain in the shadows.

We set the funeral date for the Wednesday after he died on Monday evening, which did not allow for much time to notify anyone. Clay's father and his younger daughter flew in from Tennessee, and the elder daughter and her boyfriend were already in Oklahoma City. We had reserved adjoining rooms for our families in a local motel, and Clay's Dad had adjoining rooms with his girls. Annie invited everyone to her apartment the night before the funeral. Clay's friend who lived in Guthrie, Oklahoma, brought some barbecue and grieved with the family. I think I was resting after visiting the funeral home and viewing Clay's body.

I will never get the image of Clay lying in that coffin out of my mind. He was asleep and bound in linen with an old prayer shawl around him. He looked like an 80-year old man. What a beating that young, strong body had taken! His body was at rest, but I know that his spirit was leaping around in his new home unfettered and free. My heart has never been so hollow, my soul so shriven. Is that a word? I would gladly have grieved as they do in many cultures. I needed to tear my clothes and scream with grief, to lay prostrate in my helplessness and loss. I wanted to take Clay's body in my arms and kiss his face once more. I did hold his hand and whisper my good-byes and my regrets.

Before I even got out of the hospital, I had a call from the *Long Beach Press-Telegram*. We had kept in contact with his friend Dave in Long Beach and he had let the paper know that Clay had died. Because he had been instrumental in founding Being Alive/Long Beach, a support group who helped hundreds of men who had AIDS, and was the last survivor of those co-founders, they wanted to do an article on his life. As people found out about Clay's death, they shared with me his contributions to those suffering with the disease and with the system. I felt even more humbled that I had been able to help someone who had helped so many. I headed home to write the obituary for the newspapers.

Clay would have enjoyed the gathering at his funeral. A few close friends, all of his brothers and sisters, his father and stepfather and my friends. Among those attending were his professors and colleagues from colleges who spoke words of honor for him. His professors and those who worked with him at the Hillel Foundation in Norman shared Clay's contributions to the foundation and to his classes and classmates. We tried to follow the Jewish ritual, a brief ceremony in which a Rabbi, his Hebrew professor and friend spoke to the group. And then we followed the hearse to the cemetery. A traditional Jewish burial was new to this gentile group. The tradition of lowering his coffin into the ground and his family and friends sprinkling the dirt over his coffin was an act of release for us all. We had returned him to the earth from which he came. Leaving him there was numbing. We would not see that body again.

Clay's spirit followed us the rest of that day. A sense of relief that he was free, that the ordeal was over for all of us, and that we had one more act we had promised him, led us into a sort of reunion of lives at the graveyard. All of the half brothers and sisters, step brothers and step sisters were all together, getting to know each other. Joined in grief. The other act we had promised him? A wake—a celebration. This was how we honored him. We took our exhausted bodies to a restaurant-bar and honored him with a good, old fashioned wake. Our glasses were lifted to our lost son and brother. He was free and we were left with scars and memories.

I am writing this book because Clay wanted his life to count, and because I wanted to chronicle his life in such a way that his choices, good and bad, would offer an example to others. What type of example? In my eyes, showing the progression of his life as a vibrant, handsome young man to an old sick man in less than 15 years, could be a vicarious experience to those beginning to walk that path. If somehow I could instill in others some fear, or at least some degree of awareness of how fragile life is and how quickly it can end through my witness, I would feel that Clay's life was not wasted. I took pictures throughout the years, even pictures in the hospital and in his coffin, with the intention of someday using them as a tool to get young people's attention ...... that this could happen to them. Maybe with this presentation young people would realize they are not immune to an experience like Clay's. I have hesitated because I have felt that this would somehow intrude on Clay's privacy and dignity.

I have also avoided working on his quilt for the Names Project, the wonderful movement which coordinates the quilts made my loving hands of survivors of those who have died from AIDS. Clay's friends and caregivers have urged me to let them make it. I have gathered the materials and keepsakes, but have not yet released them to the world. Release is coming with the healing. And I know this quilt that travels over the world would bring honor to Clay and his memory.

The Jewish tradition which forbids the family from placing the tombstone for at least 11 months is rooted in centuries of wisdom. We needed that time. And one year later, the rabbi and members of Emanuel Synagogue joined with us in once more releasing his soul to his God. We took another step in the healing process. Healing requires time. The pain and raw grief subside in a different time frame and different way for each person. We go on living, but we are altered. My walk through Clay's struggle with being gay and living with AIDS was a mother's walk. With time I am becoming my own person again, but my heart has a deep scar and I still cannot believe the path we took. Clay held my hand and my heart for 33 years. He brought love, life, humor and intelligence into my life and permanently changed the paths I seek.

We were not finished visiting with you, my son. We will meet you once again at the end of that long road on which you truly WALKED LIKE A MAN.

Afterword

To Clay

If I could hold you again,
My son.
I would stroke your face and hands.
I would look into your big, blue eyes
And tell you of my love and how much I miss you.

We would talk of the birds and butterflies
And listen to Mozart and talk about injustice,
And molecules and God and Allah and all of his creatures.

Oh, if I could pull you from that deep, dark grave,
I would hug you so hard
You would live.

About the Author

Ann Baker is a woman who became a wife and mother during the Beaver-Cleaver days of the 50's and 60's. The timing of each of her varied experiences in life ultimately threw her family into the midst of the gay revolution and the beginning of the AIDS epidemic. The timeline of this book give a peek into the great American way of life through four decades. At 62, she is still on the job working at "a day job", has built a little house in the woods in eastern Oklahoma, communes with nature and keeps life outside her family at arm's length.

Bibliography

The Screaming Room: A Mother's Journal of Her Son's Struggle With AIDS,
  Barbara Peabody, 288 p., 1987, Avon Publishers.

And The Band Played On: Politics, People and the AIDS Epidemic
  Randy Shilts, 1988, Penguin Books, Viking Penguin.

0-595-20159-8